Landon's Story

Landon's Story

A Family's Transplant Journey

A Grandfather's Memoir

Eldon Joines

The events and conversations in this book have been set down to the best of the author's ability, although some names and details have been changed to protect the privacy of individuals. Some dollar figures stated are not accurate but are close based on the author's memory. Some characters and scenes may be composites, again based on the authors memory.

First paperback edition April 2021

Cover and interior book design by Eldon Joines

Cover photo by Whitney Gray
https://www.whitneygrayphotography.com/

ISBN 978-1-7368002-0-1 (paperback)
ISBN 978-1-7368002-1-8 (ebook)

Published by Joines Media
101 Swimming Hole Lane
Sparta, NC 28675
www.joinesmedia.com

For more visit www.landonsstory.com

Dedicated to my grandson Landon Allen Joines.
I pray God will continue to bless your life.

Prologue

I am not a professional writer. My wife, Kathy, and I made our living operating a small upholstery shop and fabric store in our hometown – Sparta, North Carolina. My ancestors were farmers and watermen on the Eastern Shore of Virginia by the mid-1600s, pioneers in Appalachia by the late 1700s. We have remained a close-knit family for succeeding generations. Most of us are Baptist, and we involve ourselves in our rural mountain communities. I was a Boy Scout leader for almost twenty-five years. I am a small-town native with traditional American values.

For the last forty years, I have been a genealogist and family historian for the Joines, Joynes, Jines families now spread across America. In that way, I have documented lives. When Landon, my grandson, became critically ill from the moment of his birth, the doctors told us he would die. But God revealed to us that Landon could survive with a rare small intestine transplant. Our family rallied in soul demanding ways as Landon's suffering tested our faith. With the deepest humility, I felt called upon to share our story as a written testimony of our long struggle and how God saved Landon.

Our story is told in simple terms as we lived it. The tone is what you might expect a grateful grandfather to use in telling you about the events around our living room coffee table. As a non-professional writer, it took me more than three years to complete the book manuscript. Reliving Landon's struggle is emotional and difficult. But have faith as you read. God has given us a happy ending.

Landon

The focus of so many prayers,
he might have levitated through life,
the child of repeat miracles,
the favorite boy of angels.

How many hands were touched by him?
How many lives were saved by him?
What will he recall of these things?
How will he deal with specialness?

Unto us is given a son
to proclaim all life as sacred.
This is our holy commandment,
to raise him up in compassion.

Families are deep-rooted trees
that serve untold generations.
They must endure cruel circumstances
to continue in wisdom's quest.

Each generation cites its hero.
In the clan of the family Joines
in the Blue Ridge Carolina mountains
a magnificent child endured,
and the legend of Landon was born.

by Monty Joynes

www.montyjoynes.com

Contents

Chapter 1

Birth

My last grandson, Landon Allen Joines, didn't wait until his planned delivery time. Instead, he made a rather grand entrance. Doctors had scheduled surgery to deliver him at 8:00 a.m. on April 20, 2009. His mother, Shelly, went into labor the night before.

Our landline rang at 3:00 a.m. I awoke. Kathy, my wife, picked up the receiver. "Okay, we'll be there as quick as we can." She placed her hand on my shoulder. "Get out of bed. Shelly is in labor. Jeremiah is rushing her to the hospital in Statesville. We need to get there."

It was too risky for Shelly to deliver a baby naturally. Difficult labor during her last pregnancy resulted in an emergency cesarean section. She was not supposed to go into labor. Her uterine scar could rupture. What's wrong? I felt a rush of adrenalin. My heart raced.

We jumped out of bed, got dressed, and headed for Statesville, North Carolina, about an hour away.

During the drive, Kathy called our daughter, Jessica. "Can you come this early? Will you pick up your grandmother? We want her there for Landon's birth. I'll call her and tell her to get ready." She closed her phone and turned to me, "Jessica needs to bring the boys. She'll bring your mother also."

"Good, I'm happy Mom will be there. Landon's birth could be the last birth she's there to witness. I hope she can still remember it a week from now."

For the past few months, Mom had experienced symptoms of Alzheimer's disease.

Kathy looked at the speedometer, "You better slow down or you're going to get a speeding ticket."

"I know," I said, easing my foot off the accelerator, "but we've got to get there for our grandson's birth."

"We won't get there in time if you get stopped for speeding."

True, but we needed to get there.

I didn't get a ticket, but driving to the wrong hospital didn't help. I didn't know there were two hospitals near Statesville and wouldn't listen when Kathy tried to tell me.

We did eventually arrive at the birth Hospital, getting there at about 4:30 a.m. and rushed to the maternity ward, thinking we were too late. Our timing was perfect.

Jeremiah emerged from the delivery room with the

unmistakable grin of a new father. He gave us the good news—the doctor delivered Landon a few minutes earlier. The surgery went well; mom, baby, and dad were all okay. Kathy hugged Jeremiah, then wiped her eyes. I gave him a hug and a big fatherly smile of approval. Landon's older brothers—fifteen-year-old Roger and eight-year-old Ezekiel—who had come to the hospital with their parents gathered around and beamed with smiles at the news.

Kathy asked Jeremiah, "When can we see him?"

"Soon. When the nurses get him cleaned, it will take them a few minutes. There were dark fluids in the amniotic sac. But the doctor said everything is okay—nothing to worry about. The nurses will bring him to the nursery. You can see him through those windows." He pointed at the large windows down the hall.

Our son, with the brightest smile on his face I've ever seen, gave his mother another hug and returned to the recovery room.

Kathy, our two grandsons, and I walked to the nursery. We gazed through the windows at the newborn babies. I read the nametags on the cribs—no Landon Allen Joines. I turned around and saw a waiting room across the hall from the nursery windows. We entered and sat.

Jessica arrived with her two boys—ten-year-old Gavin and three-year-old Braiden—and my mother just as Jeremiah returned and appeared in the doorway to the waiting room. He looked in, "Here comes Landon."

We rushed to the window. A nurse stood on the other side, holding Landon in her arms. She raised him to the window for us to see. He looked healthy. And, with a hint of red in the little hair he had. Roger and Ezekiel stood in front and gazed at their new little brother.

"Ooh, he's beautiful," Kathy said.

My chest swelled. I doubt anyone could tell, yet I could feel it. Another grandchild. My fifth. I counted myself among the many blessed grandfathers. I thought of Jeremiah and how he watched the birth of his son. And of Shelly, who endured labor pains and then surgery.

My mother raised her right hand and pointed her index finger toward the heavens. "Thank you, God."

Ezekiel said, "Finally, I get to be a big brother." Kathy smiled and hugged Ezekiel.

An intense feeling of love washed over me. I experienced the same emotion after I witnessed the births of my children.

Yet, with the births of my son and daughter, fear accompanied the love. It's a big responsibility to take care of and provide for a child. I had questioned if I was up to the task and proved I was by enduring sleepless nights and long days at work. But I did it.

With Landon's birth, I didn't experience fear and anxiety. Someone else would stay awake at night and tend to the little one. Not me. I could enjoy the moment and time with my grandson.

I felt a tightness in my throat. Tears welled. "Here is a member of the next generation."

I looked at my wife. I could tell she felt the same way. I put my arm around her, and she rested her head on my shoulder.

Jeremiah returned to the recovery room to comfort his wife. Before he left, he said the nurses gave Shelly medicine for the pain that would also help her relax. The nurses would move her to a room soon.

In the nursery, a nurse placed Landon in an incubator and at the back of the room. For the next few hours, we watched the pediatric nurses tend to Landon. Kathy remarked several times, "They should bring him to the windows where we can get a better look at him." The nurses didn't seem ready to do that. We took pictures, as best we could, from a distance.

At 10:00 a.m., everything seemed fine, so I decided to head back to our home in Sparta. I had work to do. The day before, I'd driven a church bus home from a Cub Scout trip to Charleston, South Carolina. I wanted to clean the bus and get it back to the church.

Kathy stayed at the hospital. She wanted to spend as much time as possible with Landon. I would return later in the evening, for more time with our new grandson, and to take Kathy home.

During my drive, I turned the volume up on the radio and sang along to every song. I celebrated the successful birth of another grandson and daydreamed about all the cool things, as a granddad, I would get to teach and show Landon.

Our home, located in the Blue Ridge Mountains of North Carolina, is across the Eastern Continental divide. It was hard to leave a newborn grandson, but it felt good to get back on the mountain.

Our homeplace is secluded. A couple of cousins live a few hundred yards to our north. To our east, south, and west, it's almost a mile to our nearest neighbors. A small river runs through our property. As a boy, I spent most of my summers wading, fishing, swimming in the river, and hunting in the surrounding forest. I knew Landon would enjoy visiting us here, as had all my grandsons.

At home, I grabbed a broom, a bucket of water, a clean cloth, and went to work on the bus. An hour into cleaning and almost finished, my cell phone rang—Kathy.

Her voice cracked, "Something is wrong with Landon. His stomach is swelling, and the doctor thinks he's losing blood. They have called for an ambulance from Baptist Hospital to come and get him. Jeremiah and Roger will go with Landon. I'll stay here with Shelly and Ezekiel. You need to get to Winston-Salem as soon as you can."

Sweat popped out on my forehead. Chill bumps covered my arms.

A transfer to Baptist Hospital meant one thing—Landon was in serious trouble.

Chapter 2

Pregnant

Sometimes things happen in a person's life. Something comes out of left field, totally unexpected. An accident. An injury. The loss of an income. That's where Jeremiah and Shelly were when she became pregnant for the third time.

My son and daughter-in-law had not planned to have another child. Not that the pregnancy was bad news, it just wasn't expected. Providing for and keeping up with their two sons was hard enough. Another child would make it more difficult.

Bills were due. Cars needed fixing. Providing food, clothing, and shelter for the young family consumed most of Jeremiah and Shelly's time and money, but they worked together to make it happen.

Roger, Shelly's firstborn and Jeremiah's stepson, was a junior in high school. Already an accomplished guitar player, he played in a band with several other teenage musicians. The band played local gigs and parties, despite none of the boys having a driver's license. Jeremiah and Shelly provided transportation and worked as roadies.

Their other son, nine-year-old Ezekiel, played football. Because the team practiced a couple of evenings each week, Jeremiah and Shelly took turns picking him up. Games were on Saturday, and I don't recall either parent ever missing a game.

Jeremiah worked in construction, and his job required heavy lifting. Backaches were common. A fall from the 2nd story of a townhouse contributed to a period of prolonged back pain for my son.

Sometime later, he obtained a general contractor's license and opened a construction company. Despite the backaches, Jeremiah continued to do a lot of physical labor.

Several years passed. The occasional back stiffness became chronic back pain. Occasionally, the problem made it too difficult for Jeremiah to work, and the family income suffered.

Shelly did her best to help with the finances. For two years, before getting pregnant with Landon, she worked as a part-time waitress for a major chain restaurant. Several months before the birth, she took a full-time position at the restaurant, hoping to make as much money as possible before the baby came. Almost nine years had passed since the birth of her last son. She longed to hold a newborn again.

Shelly and Jeremiah decided a third child would make the

family complete. Shelly instructed her doctor to do a tubal ligation during the scheduled C-section. For now, she focused on the growing baby bump.

Late in the first trimester of the pregnancy, the obstetrician scheduled an ultrasound. The doctor wanted to monitor the baby's growth. The rest of us wanted to know the sex of the baby. Jeremiah went with Shelly to the appointment.

Kathy and I, at work in our fabric store and upholstery business, expected a call. Our phone rang, and I answered.

"Do you want to know the sex of the baby?" Jeremiah said.

"Wait, let me get your mother." I opened the door to the workshop and motioned for Kathy to come to the phone.

"Okay, son. I've got you on speakerphone. What is it?"

"A boy."

Kathy jumped, then clapped. With a big smile on her face and teary eyes, she raised her hands above her head. "It's a boy."

Another grandson. Our last.

Kathy and I speculated while we waited for Shelly to choose a name.

She spent months scouring books on baby names. After much consideration, and wanting something different, she chose Landon Allen Joines. The first name was new to the family. She chose Allen to honor an uncle who passed away when she was young.

For months before Landon's scheduled arrival, his brothers

bubbled with excitement.

With the boys ready, and the name for the baby chosen, Shelly and Jeremiah focused on the pregnancy, which didn't feel any different from the first two. All her checkups routine, Landon, active in the womb, grew. Nothing hinted at any problems. Jeremiah supported his pregnant wife and provided for the family. He tried to find a solution to his back problem.

Two months before Landon's birth, I accompanied my son on a consultation with a neurosurgeon. At an earlier visit, the doctor ordered an MRI for Jeremiah. During this visit, the neurosurgeon told us the imaging revealed the presence of calcified spurs on several vertebrae. The spurs pressed against nerves, causing the pain. The doctor said he could not remove the spurs, and he recommended a complicated surgery to fuse the vertebrae. Jeremiah needed surgery. But an obstacle stood in the way.

Recovery from surgery would be long, six months, or more. Jeremiah would be unable to work and be of little help in taking care of a newborn; not working meant no income.

The neurosurgeon, Jeremiah, and I talked about the situation. Jeremiah decided to delay the surgery until after Landon's birth. He felt having a newborn baby in the house with him recovering from back surgery would be too much for the family. And, he didn't want to put more of a burden on his wife.

The doctor agreed. He assured us he would be available to do the surgery when Jeremiah was ready. He prescribed a medication for the pain until that time.

Shelly worked as a server at the restaurant until the last month. Because of her size—huge as she has often said—she struggled to get around the dining area and stayed in the kitchen to work as an expeditor. Doing so required her to stand near the heat lamps during her shift. On several nights, feeling faint, she soaked a towel in cold water and wrapped it around her neck. Despite being uncomfortable and because the family needed the money, Shelly worked until the day before the scheduled delivery.

During the pregnancy, Jeremiah and Shelly attended birthing and parenting classes. At first, once a month, then every two weeks, and later every week, as Shelly's due date got closer. All indicators pointed to a normal birth for Landon. Shelly and her doctor scheduled the C-section. The pregnancy progressed right on track, despite Shelly struggling a little bit during the last month.

The first sign of trouble appeared when Shelly went into labor a few hours before the scheduled delivery. Kathy and I had been present for the birth of our two children and three of our grandsons. We thought Landon was just anxious to make his entrance.

God knew otherwise. What soon unfolded changed our lives. We often hear God uses everything for His good. I would have argued that before Landon's birth.

The Universe, the world, living organisms are too complex to have come into existence by coincidence. I believed in intelligent design and an intelligent designer, God. But I didn't think God took an interest in our little problems. I didn't believe in a God above, looking over us, directing our lives, or protecting us. I felt that when we encounter problems and obstacles, it's up to us to solve those problems and overcome those obstacles, without the intervention of God.

We were ready for this new creation, Landon, to enter the world.

But we didn't expect what happened next.

Chapter 3

Something is Wrong

Few things in life rival the excitement of birth. Family photos with the newborn. Tears of joy.

We experienced all of that with Landon. But the mood changed soon after I left the hospital and returned home. The family realized that something was wrong.

Now in her room, the nurses tried to keep Shelly comfortable. The new mother often asked to see her son. Each time she asked, the nurses told her she could see Landon and hold him when she felt a little better. Jeremiah and Shelly noticed the nurses became quiet around them. Worse, the nurses wouldn't make eye contact. Shelly's level of concern and agitation grew with each passing hour.

At the nursery windows, Kathy turned to Jessica. "Something's wrong."

"Why do you say that?"

"A few minutes ago, a nurse brought a newborn in and placed it right here in a crib in front of the window, yet they still have Landon in the back of the nursery. Look how pale he is. Have you noticed how he holds his knees up to his belly? He won't straighten out and lie flat."

Kathy moved back to the waiting room and tried to help Jessica entertain her energetic toddler, Braiden. Kathy held little Braiden's hand and walked him through the hallways. Afterward, she attempted to talk with her other grandsons Roger, Ezekiel, and Gavin, in a light-hearted way. Concern for Landon occupied her mind, and she often returned to the nursery windows to check on him.

My mother, confused and agitated, paced from the waiting room to the nursery windows, and back to the waiting room.

Jeremiah stayed with Shelly most of the time, only coming to the waiting room a few times to check on the family and to see if anything had changed in regard to Landon.

About 11:30 a.m., the doctor who had delivered Landon entered Shelly's room. After asking how she felt and getting a satisfactory answer, the doctor got right to the point. "Something's wrong with Landon. His abdomen is swelling. I think he is losing blood internally. We can't help him here. He needs to go to Winston-Salem. We have called for a pediatric transport team from Brenner Children's Hospital to come and get him. They will be here soon."

The gush of information flooded the room. With the fears of

the last few hours confirmed, Shelly cried, while Jeremiah tried to contain his emotions.

The doctor turned to leave.

Shelly blurted, "Can I go with Landon?"

"No," the doctor said, "you're in no condition to leave the hospital." He looked at Jeremiah. "You need to go with your son. Your wife should stay here."

"When can I go?" Shelly asked.

"Tomorrow, maybe. I'll check on you in the morning. If you're doing well, I'll discharge you."

"Can I see my son before they take him away?"

"Yes. I'll have a nurse take you to the nursery. You can hold him, and your family can go into the nursery to see him."

The doctor walked out of the room.

Shelly sobbed. Jeremiah pulled her into his arms, telling her, "Everything will be okay."

He didn't know what else to say to comfort his wife. To both, this felt like a blurry dream.

Jeremiah pulled a tissue from a box on the table beside of Shelly's bed and handed it to his wife. "I need to go tell Mom what's happening."

Kathy stood at the window to the nursery. The sudden, new activity around Landon alarmed her. She saw the fear on her son's face as he approached. He confirmed her suspicions by repeating what the doctor had said moments before.

Kathy's throat tightened and tears formed in her eyes. Jeremiah put his arms around his mother and pulled her close. The fear of the unknown overcame him. He lost it for the first time since Landon's birth. Jessica heard what her brother had said. She came over and put her arms around her mother and brother. Together they cried.

A nurse brought Shelly, in a wheelchair, to the nursery. Another nurse removed Landon from the crib and placed him in his mother's arms. Tears streamed from Shelly's eyes. She looked at her baby's face and caressed his cheek with the back of her index finger. Jeremiah, Kathy, Roger, and Ezekiel gathered around Shelly. Taking turns, kneeling, or bending, they each touched Landon's hair or rubbed his arm.

The love of the family surrounded the sick infant. He opened his beautiful blue eyes. The hint of red in his hair was even more apparent. Despite being showered with love, Landon showed signs of pain. He grimaced, and he moaned a few times.

Regardless of Shelly's eyes being red from crying, Kathy took a family picture. Shelly kissed her son's forehead, handed him to a nurse, and returned to her room.

The nurses took over and prepared Landon for the trip to Winston-Salem, a little more than forty miles away. They placed Landon in an incubator and taped leads on several places on his body. Wires connected the leads to a monitor. They inserted an IV into his right hand and started fluids and antibiotics. A nurse inserted a tube into one of his nostrils to supplement his oxygen.

She taped the tube to his face.

The sudden activity and the pace the nurses worked at alarmed Jeremiah. He realized that time had become a factor. He paced the hall, from his wife's room to the nursery windows and back to her room. He tried to comfort Shelly and, at the same time, watch what the nurses did to prepare Landon for the trip.

The day had been long for little Braiden and my mother. Jessica took them, along with Gavin, and headed home to the mountains, about fifty miles away.

The transport team from Brenner Children's Hospital soon arrived and whisked Landon away. They made a brief stop in his mother's room for her to say goodbye. She caressed her baby's hand with the tip of her finger and whispered, in a broken, tearful voice, "I love you. Get better soon."

Jeremiah and Roger followed the transport team outside and watched them load Landon into the ambulance. The two rushed to the family car and fell in behind the emergency vehicle. Lights flashing and siren blaring, the ambulance zoomed past other traffic with my son and grandson following.

As they followed the ambulance, Roger, a couple of weeks away from his sixteenth birthday, talked with Jeremiah. Jeremiah tried to lighten the mood and asked his stepson what he wanted for his birthday. The teenager mentioned a few video games, but the conversation ultimately shifted back to Landon. Roger's voice cracked at times, and Jeremiah sensed his fear. He tried to assure him that everything would be okay. "Brenner Children's Hospital is the best hospital for Landon. It won't take the doctors there long to find out what's wrong."

Kathy, Shelly, and Ezekiel remained in the hospital room.

With Landon en route to Winston-Salem and a facility better suited to care for him, in Statesville, Shelly and her recovery became the top priority.

She cried a lot, tried to watched TV, to sleep. Nothing brought comfort or peace of mind.

Kathy took Ezekiel to the hospital cafeteria to get a sandwich.

While they were gone, a nurse came to Shelly's room. She brought news. Landon had arrived at Baptist Hospital.

The nurse said, "How's the pain?"

"Not too bad. The medicine helps."

The nurse placed a thermometer under Shelly's tongue and a blood pressure cuff around her left arm. After recording the readings, the nurse asked an unusual question—for a nurse these days anyway. "Can I pray for you and your son?"

"Yes," Shelly said.

The nurse stood at the end of the bed, placed her hands on the covers over Shelly's feet, and prayed. She prayed the doctors in Winston-Salem would discover what was wrong with Landon. She prayed for his healing. She prayed for Shelly's healing and comfort. She ended the prayer with, "in the name of Jesus Christ, I pray."

Shelly looked at the nurse and smiled.

The nurse said, "I'll bring you another Sprite in a few minutes."

She left the room.

A few minutes later, Kathy and Ezekiel returned from the cafeteria, each carrying an extra-large clear plastic cup, filled with ice and Mt. Dew.

Shelly's stomach hurt. She struggled to sit upright in her bed, as she sipped Sprite from a small white Styrofoam cup.

While Shelly tried to rest and Ezekiel sat in a chair watching television, Kathy went to the hospital gift shop. She wandered through the aisles. She picked up a fuzzy blue stuffed bear with a long blue ribbon attached to it, looked at it, and thought about her little grandson. Kathy held the stuffed animal close to her chest while a tear rolled down her cheek. She purchased the bear, returned to Shelly's room, and gave it to her daughter-in-law.

Shelly hugged it, took an ink pen, and wrote Landon's name, birth date, and birth weight on the attached card then asked Kathy to hang it on a hook on the door to her room.

An hour later, a friend, Angie, showed up. "I like the bear," she said, as she entered the room.

Shelly and Angie had been friends for more than eight years. They met when they were both waitresses at Harry Gant's Steakhouse in Taylorsville, NC. Angie always had a way of cheering Shelly up. She tried on this day, but all she could get out of Shelly was a smile.

Ezekiel changed the channels on the television and turned the volume up and down. At his age, his attention span was short.

Angie said, "Let me take Ezekiel home with me. I'll feed him a good supper, and he can play video games with my two boys."

Ezekiel was all for it, and Shelly agreed.

Thirty minutes later, Angie hugged Shelly and said her goodbyes. "Call me when you hear from Jeremiah, or if you need to talk."

With Shelly's middle son gone, and the volume turned down on the television, she closed her eyes and tried to sleep. But sleep wouldn't come. Jeremiah called a couple of times, but not with any answers. Landon had been at Baptist hospital for several hours, and the doctors there still didn't know what was wrong with him.

About 5:30 p.m., Shelly's cousin Tracy arrived. Shelly was not asleep. Kathy sat in a chair on the opposite side of the bed, watching the television on the wall. Tracy leaned over Shelly's bed, hugged her, and whispered, "God will not give you more than you can bear. He is here for you."

Tears formed in Shelly's eyes. She shook her head in agreement, "Thank you. I needed to hear that."

Kathy had a problem. She wanted to go to Baptist Hospital early the next morning, but she didn't have a vehicle. Jeremiah and Shelly owned a second vehicle, so Kathy asked Tracy to take her to Jeremiah and Shelly's home to get it.

Tracy offered other support too. The next day was her day off from work. She would come to the birth hospital early in the morning and stay with Shelly. If the doctor agreed to discharge Shelly, she would drive her to Baptist Hospital. Tracy and Kathy left the birth hospital at about 6:30 p.m. For the first time that day,

Shelly was alone.

She was talking on the phone when two coworkers arrived.

"Jennifer and Paul are here. I'll call you back when they leave." She hung up the phone.

Jennifer leaned over and hugged Shelly. Paul placed a gift basket on the table beside the bed.

"How are you?" Jennifer asked.

Shelly said, "Okay, I guess, a little sore."

Paul said, "How's the little one? This afternoon we heard that something's wrong. You know how it is, news travels fast at the restaurant."

"That was Jeremiah on the phone," Shelly said. "We still don't know what's wrong."

She tried not to cry in front of her friends. The two stayed for about forty-five minutes.

Before they left, Paul said, "Let us know as soon as you find out what's wrong."

"I will," Shelly said.

They left at about 7:30 p.m.

Thirty minutes later, Shelly's mother, Susan, arrived. Through a steady stream of tears, the daughter filled her mother in on what had happened.

Susan said, "Shelly, I wish I could stay the night with you, but

I have to work tomorrow. I can't get off."

"That's okay. There's been a constant flow of visitors all day. It's wearing me out. I'm going to try to sleep when you leave."

Susan stayed for about an hour. At home, she called her parents, Herman and Doris, and told them what had happened with Landon, and about their granddaughter, alone, at the hospital in Statesville.

Shelly's grandparents, both devout Christians, attended Stony Point Baptist Church. Herman called their pastor and asked him to visit Shelly the next morning at the hospital in Statesville. The pastor said he had a full schedule for the next day. However, he promised to visit Shelly first.

A little past midnight, the phone in Shelly's room rang. Jeremiah. They talked for a few minutes.

Before saying goodbye, Shelly said, "Call me if you find out anything. Call me as often as you can. I'm going crazy here. I need to hear your voice."

I couldn't imagine a day filled with more emotion than this day had been. For Shelly, it started with labor pains. Our family experienced the excitement and joy of Landon's birth. Love washed over us when we first saw his beautiful face. Concern and fear crept in as we realized something was wrong. Sorrow overtook us as the transport team wheeled him away.

Now, Shelly could only imagine what was happening to her baby, fifty miles away.

Chapter 4

The Long Night

My head spun. Questions flashed in my mind. How is he losing blood? Why is his belly swelling? Landon seemed fine when I left the hospital in Statesville a few hours ago. What happened? The doctors in Winston-Salem, fifty miles away, would have answers. I had to get there.

On Highway 21, with Kathy not there to slow me, I descended the Blue Ridge Escarpment. Around the curves, the two-door sedan handled like Jeff Gordon's Chevrolet at Watkins Glen. Tires squealed. At the bottom of the mountain, I lowered the driver's side window. Cool, springtime air rushed into the car. Sweat evaporated from my face, and my head cleared. Confidence blended with my sense of urgency.

After my grandson Braiden's birth, three years earlier, he had trouble breathing. The doctors at his birth hospital transferred him to Baptist Hospital, where they diagnosed the problem, treated him, and sent him home a few days later. Confident the doctors at Baptist would do the same for Landon; I drove on.

Having been there before, I knew how to get to Wake Forest Baptist Medical Center. I entered the parking deck and found a space several floors up.

I called Jeremiah's cell phone. He didn't answer.

Exiting the vehicle, I called Kathy. "Where's Jeremiah?"

"I talked to him a few minutes ago." she said, "They are taking Landon to the Neonatal Intensive Care Unit, the NICU. You need to go there."

I grabbed a light fleece jacket from my car, trotted to the main entrance, entered through large glass doors, approached an information desk, then paused to catch my breath.

"Can I help you?" the woman seated behind the desk said.

"Where's the NICU?"

"Take the elevator to the fourth floor."

She seemed to know what my next question would be and pointed to a sign across the room. Elevators. An arrow pointed towards a hallway. I nodded. In the hall, I found Jeremiah and Roger at the entrance to a room with a bank of elevators.

My son's pale face made him look sick.

Red-eyed and out of breath, he spoke fast. His voice cracked, "We are following Landon to the NICU."

Two male nurses, each with a hand on Landon's incubator, waited for an elevator to open.

Landon, wrapped in a blue blanket, did not move. He looked peaceful. But, after seeing Jeremiah so shaken, my concern ramped up considerably.

A door opened. The nurses pushed the incubator on to the elevator, and we followed.

Inside, I asked my son more questions. He told me what happened in Statesville, after I left, and described the trip to Winston-Salem.

I shivered, slipped my arms into the fleece jacket, and tried to reassure Jeremiah. "Son, this is the best hospital around. The doctors here will find out what's wrong and fix the problem soon."

At the entrance to the NICU, a woman, seated behind a counter, pressed a button. The doors to the NICU opened. The two men pushed Landon's incubator through the doors.

The woman said, "The daddy can go back with the baby." She looked at me then pointed at a waiting room across the hall, "Y'all can have a seat in there."

She smiled—the gatekeeper. No one entered the NICU without her approval.

Jeremiah entered.

Roger and I found seats at the back of the waiting room. I tried to assimilate the information my son had given me and hoped the doctors would diagnose the problem soon.

An hour passed. What were the doctors doing? I needed to talk to Jeremiah.

I should be allowed in the NICU. He's my grandson, but the "gatekeeper" said no.

Even so, she had a happy cackle that echoed through the corridors while she swapped stories and joked with a security guard.

I walked into the hallway, looked in both directions, then looked at the woman behind the counter. Her face did not reflect her jovial laughter. She stared back at me with a glare that said, "Don't even think about it." I returned to my seat.

Finally, Jeremiah emerged from the NICU. "What time is it?"

"Three-thirty," I said.

"I need to call Shelly. You can go back to see Landon."

"First, son, tell me what's happening. Has the doctor seen Landon? Have they found anything? What are they doing?"

"A doctor came to see Landon when we first arrived. He asked me to describe the birth and what happened in Statesville. He said Landon's hemoglobin is low. The nurses are giving him blood, and they drew blood for testing. The results should be back soon."

"Good. It sounds like the doctors and nurses are doing what they need to do. We'll know what's wrong soon."

Jeremiah called Shelly.

I approached the woman at the counter. "I need to go in to

see Landon Joines."

"And who are you?"

"I'm his grandfather."

She picked up the phone receiver on her desk. "Can Landon Joines' papaw come back to see him?" A moment later, she smiled, pressed the button, and the doors opened.

A nurse met me at the entrance and showed me where to find my grandson.

No longer in an incubator, he lay in a crib, a metal table on wheels with a small—baby size—mattress on top of it. Clear plexiglass, about a quarter-inch thick and eight inches high, surrounded him.

The sight of this baby boy overwhelmed me. He slept, covered with the little blue blanket. Wires emerged from under the covers and connected to a monitor hanging on a pole. Clear plastic tubes dangled from bags hung on poles and carried fluids into his little veins. A blue knitted toboggan covered the top of his head.

His little hand looked tiny in my palm while my fingers gently closed around it. My right hand covered the top of his head and the fuzzy toboggan. An urge to pick him up and hold him close came over me. I didn't but choked back tears, content to gaze at him and touch him.

I looked at the monitor beside his bed and tried to make sense of the information on the screen. Did it indicate anything unusual? I couldn't determine.

I stayed with Landon for about an hour, then returned to the waiting room. Jeremiah, Roger, and I waited there for another hour.

A young doctor wearing a white coat emerged from the NICU. He approached us and sat beside Jeremiah. "We still don't know what's wrong with your son. What few test results we have, don't show anything. I have ordered several other tests. It shouldn't take long to get the results back. We'll continue to give him blood and antibiotics." He stood. "My shift will be over soon. Another doctor will be out to talk to you when we know more."

The doctor returned to the NICU in a hurry, not giving us time to ask any questions.

Jeremiah, still sitting in a chair, tilted his head back. He placed the palms of his hands on his forehead then dragged them down his face, over the stubble, until his fingertips stopped on his chin. He looked at the ceiling. "We've been here almost five hours, and we still don't know any more than we did when we got here. What can we do?" He leaned forward, placed his elbows on his knees, and his face in his hands.

I put my left arm around his shoulder, "All we can do is wait. The doctors are doing all they can. We'll know something soon." I wasn't so sure, but what else could we do? I didn't consider praying.

It was getting late, and we were hungry, but we didn't want to go far from the waiting room in case the doctor came out with an update. I found a snack machine and bought crackers and drinks for the three of us. We sat in silence, nibbled, and stared at the TV.

An hour later, Jeremiah returned to the NICU. I stayed in the waiting room. Roger played video games.

I closed my eyes. My mind flashed to Landon and the scene inside the NICU. How much longer?

About 10:30 p.m., I called Kathy, "We don't know anything yet. I'll call you if the doctors find something during the night."

"I'll sleep on the sofa here at Jeremiah's house," Kathy said. "Tomorrow morning, I'll come to Winston. Kiss Landon for me."

A few minutes before midnight, an older doctor, balding with short gray hair around the sides, came into the waiting room. He became Landon's doctor after the shift change five hours earlier. He carried a clipboard in one hand and a pen in the other. Jeremiah had returned from the NICU a few minutes earlier. The doctor sat in a chair across from us.

"I think Landon's liver is bleeding."

"How could his liver be bleeding?" I said. "What could have caused that to happen?"

"Something might have happened during birth," the doctor said. "Maybe a doctor or nurse roughly handled Landon. It doesn't happen often, but it is possible."

Jeremiah said, "I watched Landon's birth. I don't remember anyone handling him roughly. I took a video. I can show it to you."

He pulled his phone from his pocket.

"No, you don't need to," the doctor said. "If a nurse or doctor didn't injure him during the birth, maybe something injured him before his birth." He looked at Jeremiah, "Did your wife take a fall recently?"

"No."

"Did your wife get hit in the abdomen?"

Jeremiah looked offended. "Doctor, if you're suggesting I hit my wife and injured my son, the answer is no. I don't hit my wife."

"Okay, I had to ask. In any case, we need to get a scan of your son's liver. I have called for a technician to come and do an ultrasound. When the tech gets here, the nurses will take Landon to the exam room." The doctor leaned forward. "Landon's temperature has risen. His blood pressure is unstable. We may not have much more time to figure out what's wrong. Is there anything else you can tell me about your son's birth? Anything unusual?"

"I've already mentioned the dark fluids. There's nothing else," Jeremiah said.

The doctor scribbled a note on the clipboard, placed the ink pen in his shirt pocket, and stood. He and Jeremiah shook hands before the doctor returned to the NICU.

Jeremiah called Shelly.

The doctor didn't give us any new information, so I didn't call Kathy.

The clock ticked well past midnight. We were tired but couldn't sleep. When I closed my eyes, they popped right back open.

About 1:30 a.m., the door to the NICU opened. Two female nurses emerged, pushing Landon in his crib. One of them motioned for us to follow.

Roger watched a muted late-night show on the television and stayed in the waiting room.

Jeremiah and I followed the nurses through a long narrow hallway to an exam room. They pushed the crib through a door then instructed the two of us to remain outside in the hall.

With no place to sit, and too tired to stand, we slumped to the floor and leaned against the wall.

Several minutes later, one of the nurses came to the door. "We can't get a needle into Landon's veins. We've tried several times. We've asked a transport nurse to come here from the emergency room to give it a try. She works with little collapsed veins all the time. Maybe she'll be able to get the needle in."

My son and I remained seated on the floor.

Jeremiah couldn't sit still. Turning from side to side, he said, "My back hurts bad, but I don't want to take anything that will make me drowsy."

"Son, when we get back to the waiting room, you need to stretch out and relax. I'll sit with Landon."

"No," Jeremiah said, "I want to stay with my son. There's a recliner in the NICU. I can put it beside Landon's crib. I'll rest better there."

The transport nurse arrived. Within a few minutes, she inserted a needle in a vein.

In less than thirty minutes, the technician completed the ultrasound.

The nurses pushed the crib out of the exam room.

One of the nurses looked at us while we rose from the floor, "His blood pressure is low. He needs fluids. We've got to get him back to the NICU fast."

They rushed through the empty hallways pushing the crib. The sound of hurried footsteps on tile floors and a squeaky wheel echoed through the halls. I tried to keep up. My heart thumped in my throat and pounded in my ears.

At the NICU, Jeremiah entered behind the nurses.

I stopped in the hall, gasped for air, and looked at my phone, 3:00 a.m., twenty-four hours since a telephone woke me.

In the waiting room, Roger had curled into a fetal position on a chair. He slept. The lights were off. I slipped into the dim room and sat in a chair in the back corner. My heartbeat slowed to a steady thumping in my chest. I pulled my fleece jacket over my shoulders and closed my eyes.

My thoughts bounced from Landon to Jeremiah, to Shelly, to Kathy, and back to Landon. Always back to Landon.

My grandson arrived at this hospital more than fourteen hours earlier—still, we had no answers. The images of him in the crib, fighting for his life, crushed my heart.

Will the doctors figure out what's wrong before it's too late?

My swirling mind drained what little energy I had left. Finally, I dozed.

Chapter 5

Blockage

I had faith in doctors. Medical schools train physicians to figure out what's wrong, treat, and heal sick patients. The doctors used a process of elimination while they tried to figure out what was wrong. A difficult undertaking because little Landon could not tell the doctors where he hurt. But he gave clues. He drew his legs to his abdomen, he grimaced. They ordered several tests. When those didn't reveal the problem, they ordered more tests. We waited.

Jeremiah touched my shoulder. He spoke. I shook my head, sat, and looked around. Where was I? The cobwebs cleared. My thoughts connected. Landon. Hospital. Waiting room.

"It's seven o'clock," Jeremiah said, "you need to come with me."

I had slept for almost four hours. I rose, the waking-up fog almost gone.

"We need to meet a doctor in the NICU in a few minutes," he said. "She wants to talk to us."

"Is Landon okay?"

"Yes, after we got him back to the NICU last night, the nurses connected more fluids, and his blood pressure stabilized."

"Good," I said.

Inside the NICU, a doctor we hadn't seen before and five young people, all dressed in white coats, huddled in the walkway a few feet from my grandson. We walked to Landon's crib, stood, and watched the group.

Wake Forest Baptist Medical Center is a teaching hospital. Maybe this young doctor and her bright pupils can figure out what's wrong with my grandson.

The medical team whispered amongst themselves, yet loud enough that I caught a word now and then. Hemoglobin. Fever. Abdomen. The doctor, a thin woman, several inches shorter than me, and about thirty years old, had olive-colored skin, dark eyes, and long brown hair. Her small stature, dark skin, and long hair made her appear Middle Eastern or of Indian descent. She led the conversation and waved her hands to describe something to the team.

The doctor and the physicians-in-training walked over to Landon's crib and surrounded us. She introduced herself and her associates. Making eye contact with a couple of students, she pointed to one of the monitors. The doctor reached into Landon's crib, adjusted the small blue blanket, touched his forehead, and then his cheeks, with the back of her hand.

She seemed energetic yet nervous. "Landon is a sick little boy and getting sicker. We don't have much time to figure out what's wrong with him."

I said, "What about the liver scan? Did it show anything?"

"No," the doctor said. "There's nothing wrong with his liver. None of the tests have revealed anything. Nothing that could make Landon this sick."

"So, what's wrong?" Jeremiah said, a look of frustration on his face.

The doctor said, "I noticed you mentioned the dark fluids present at his birth. That might have been bile, a result of bilious vomiting. There's another test we need to do. We need to get a look at his stomach and intestine. We need to run a tube with a camera on it down his throat. I will order an upper GI. A technician will do it as soon as we can get your son into the lab."

I sensed a high level of confidence in this doctor's voice.

I glanced at Jeremiah. He looked worried, tired.

Jeremiah and I returned to the NICU waiting room. I sat beside my son and said, "I feel good about this doctor. She's a take-charge kind of person."

"What could an upper GI show us?"

"I don't know. Maybe Landon's bleeding from his stomach. If this doesn't show anything, at least they will have eliminated another possibility."

After Jeremiah called Shelly, he returned to the NICU to sit with his son.

I called Kathy.

"I've already left Jeremiah's house," she said. "I'll be there within the hour."

Roger had been asleep in the waiting room. Now awake, I asked him to come with me to the hospital cafeteria.

Roger came into our lives when he was three years old. Kathy and I loved him and treated him like a biological grandson. He had been a good big brother to Ezekiel. That might explain why Ezekiel wanted to be a big brother—brotherly love.

Roger and I walked through the halls, rode the elevator, and talked.

It could have been puberty or emotion, but the pitch in Roger's voice changed while we discussed his little brother. He asked about the upcoming test and how much longer I thought we might be at the hospital.

"The doctors will find out what's wrong soon." I'm not sure if my words convinced him. My confidence wavered, sort of like Roger's voice.

We brought our breakfast back to the NICU waiting room. Roger turned on the television while I stared out of the windows. Outside, a beautiful spring morning unfolded. Dogwoods bloomed. Inside, my faith wilted, and my patience dried.

About 9:30 a.m., Jeremiah, Roger, and I followed the doctor and her entourage through a hallway to an exam room. The medical team pushed the crib with Landon inside, into the room.

The doctor instructed us to stay in the hallway. Again, we waited. And still, no place to sit.

Jeremiah said, "Boy, last night was brutal. My back hurts this morning."

We leaned against the walls.

Jeremiah's stomach rumbled. I turned to asked if he wanted me to get him something to eat. The doors to the examination room flew open and smacked the wall.

Landon's doctor stood there with her eyes the size of fifty-cent pieces. She looked at Jeremiah. "We found it. He has a blockage in his intestine. He needs surgery. We've got to get to the operating room. When the surgeon gets here, we will begin."

Blood drained from my face, followed by a massive surge of adrenalin.

The doctor looked at Jeremiah. "Come with us to the operating room." She pointed at Roger and me. "Go to the surgical waiting room."

The doctor moved to one side, and the medical team swooshed passed, pushing Landon's crib. The doctor followed.

Jeremiah ran behind. After six or eight steps, he turned and shouted, "I'll call Shelly."

Even from a distance, I could see the fear on my son's face.

I shouted back, "I'll call your mom. We'll be in the waiting room. Let us know when they begin the...." A lump formed in my throat. I couldn't finish the sentence. Jeremiah was too far down the hall to hear me anyway.

Surgery. Something I hadn't considered. The doctors discovered the problem. They found a blockage. Fix it. Do the surgery. Heal our grandson. My thoughts turned to my wife.

With a trembling finger, I pressed the number for Kathy. "They found something," I paused to catch my breath. "Where are you?"

"I'm almost there. Where should I go?"

A few minutes later, Roger and I met Kathy at the main entrance. The three of us followed the signs to the surgical waiting room.

The waiting area consisted of two rooms, a large one that we entered directly into from the hall and a smaller one to the left of the big room. With scheduled surgeries underway, only a few unoccupied seats remained. We found chairs at the far end of the large room, under a row of windows. After I gave Kathy an update, she called Jessica and asked our daughter to pick up my mother and get here as soon as she could.

Thirty minutes later, Jeremiah entered the waiting room. He hugged his mother. "Landon is in a pre-op room. When the pediatric surgeon gets here, Landon will get the next available operating room. His surgery is an emergency. He will get top priority. Shelly checked herself out of the hospital in Statesville a few minutes ago. She and Tracy will be here soon. Angie is on her way with Ezekiel."

Jeremiah returned to the pre-op room, and I went to the cafeteria for a cup of coffee.

When I came back, I discovered Angie and Ezekiel had arrived. Kathy and Angie sat together, as did the brothers. The family was gathering.

A few minutes passed. Jeremiah returned from the pre-op room. His eyes wide with excitement, he spoke fast, "They have taken Landon to the operating room. Shelly just got here. I'm on my way to meet them. I'll hurry. I don't know how long the surgery will take."

Roger, Ezekiel, and Angie followed Jeremiah to meet Shelly and Tracy. Kathy stayed with me.

While we discussed the surgery, I overheard a man ask the woman at the information counter, "Is the Landon Joines family here?"

I stood, walked over, and extended my hand, "I'm Landon's grandfather."

The broad-shouldered man, who wore a white shirt, tie, and suit jacket, grabbed my hand with a firm grip and shook it. "I'm the pastor of Stony Point Baptist Church. Shelly's grandparents are members."

"Did Shelly's grandfather ask you to come here?"

"No, he asked me to go to Statesville. When I got there, they told me Shelly left a few minutes earlier to go to Winston-Salem for her baby's emergency surgery. I decided to go back to Stony Point, but at the interstate, I suddenly felt I should come here. How's the baby?"

Before I could answer, the doors to the operating room opened. Several doctors emerged, and I recognized one, the female doctor from the NICU. I scanned their faces. The look of urgency sent ripples of panic through my body.

One of the doctors, in a loud voice, said, "Joines Family?"

I raised my hand. "I'm Landon's grandfather."

"Where are his parents?"

Again, before I could answer, another door opened, the one from the hallway to the waiting room. Shelly, in a wheelchair, came through. Jeremiah pushed the chair. Tracy, Angie, Roger, and Ezekiel followed.

The doctor looked at all of us. "Follow me."

He led us into a small, rectangle conference room. The medical team entered first. Chairs lined the walls, but no one sat. Our family stood on the left side of the room and faced the doctors on the right. Kathy, on my left, wrapped her arms around Ezekiel's shoulders. To my right, Jeremiah held the handles of Shelly's wheelchair. Tracy and Angie stood on the other side of Shelly. Beyond them, Roger and the pastor in a corner.

A balding doctor, fortyish, tall, thin, dressed in blue scrubs, spoke in a soft, slow manner, "I'm a pediatric surgeon. I operated on Landon. I found your son's intestine twisted. It had twisted around the artery that supplies blood to the small intestine. The twisting cut off the blood to his intestine. The medical term is malrotation with midgut volvulus."

I studied his face. Solemn, sympathetic, compassionate.

"Landon's small intestine appears dead, all of it." He paused.

The words sank in. I placed my hand over my mouth and held my breath. Silence, shattered by the doctor's next words, "A person cannot live without a small intestine. Landon is going to die."

Chapter 6

Waiting for Death

"Landon is going to die," reverberated through the small conference room.

"No, no," I said. The words came from somewhere deep inside. Visceral. Like a punch in the gut.

I had planned so much for this grandson—camping, hiking, fishing. Now, the dream, his life, over before it even started.

With my left arm around my wife, I leaned forward. Tears dripped from my cheeks.

Kathy, crying, placed her hand over Ezekiel's ear then pulled his head to her breast, shielding him from the words that hung in the room.

Jeremiah stood frozen, gripping the handles on Shelly's wheelchair, his knuckles white. He focused on the surgeon then blinked. Tears gushed from his eyes and fell on Shelly's back.

Shelly, head lowered, sobbed, heaved, and sobbed more.

Roger wept.

The pastor—Roger's previous youth minister—held him, "I've got you, Roger."

The doctor's sympathetic looks. Moist eyes.

Several minutes passed. Sniffles. Sobs. I wiped tears with my palms—snot with my shirt sleeves.

The surgeon said, "We have untwisted Landon's intestine and taped his abdomen closed. Tomorrow morning, we will have another look to see if there is any sign of blood flow. I don't expect that to happen. We will take Landon back to the NICU. All of you can see him there."

"How long?" I asked.

The doctor, hesitant, quiet for several seconds, said, "It's tough to say. Forty-eight hours, maybe seventy-two. No more."

Two days, three days at the most, and my grandson would be dead.

The pastor said, "Can I pray for Landon?"

"Absolutely," I said.

Jeremiah, eyes still fixed on the surgeon, nodded.

The pastor prayed, "Our heavenly Father, we will accept Your will. If it is Your will this little child shall die, we will accept it. Your will be done. But Lord, we ask for a miracle. This family wants this baby to live. We pray for You to save little Landon. In the name of Jesus Christ, we pray. Amen"

A little before noon, we filed out of the conference room. The medical team went back to the operating rooms. Our family held each other, wiped away tears, and walked through the crowded waiting room.

Ezekiel turned to his grandmother. "Does this mean I can't be a big brother?"

Mascara streaked Kathy's face. She wrapped her arm around Ezekiel's shoulders.

The previous twenty-four hours had been about solving a mystery. Now, we had the answer.

Not what we hoped for—not death. We expected the doctors to find the problem and fix it. They couldn't. No hope. Now, they gave us a place to sit, say goodbye to our baby, and watch him die.

At the NICU, nurses brought Landon back from the operating room.

The original gatekeeper had retaken command of the unit. She recognized Jeremiah, opened the door, and he wheeled Shelly in.

The rest of us entered the waiting room. No one spoke. We sat, wiped away tears, sniffled, and waited for our time to say goodbye.

In the NICU, a nurse placed Landon in Shelly's arms and

pulled a tall folding privacy screen around the grieving couple and their baby. Jeremiah knelt beside the wheelchair and wrapped his arms around his wife and little boy. The nurses left them alone in their grief. They remained with their son for more than an hour. Then came our turn.

The sight of him stopped us in our tracks. Kathy held her hand over her mouth to keep from sobbing out loud. Ten feet from his crib, my wife and I held each other, cried, and looked at our grandson.

Landon lay flat on his back. His body swollen. A ventilator tube in his mouth. IVs in his arms and hands. A piece of white tape held a tube in his nose. An orange bandage covered his distended abdomen. His face puffy, his eyes red, he didn't look like the same little boy we saw the day before.

Kathy approached first, stood beside his crib, held his right hand, and stared at his little face. I stood on the other side of the crib and took pictures with a small digital camera.

In the waiting room, Jessica, her two boys, and my mother arrived.

Jeremiah approached the woman at the counter and asked if he could take his grandmother in to see Landon.

The woman, a look of sympathy and sorrow on her face, said, "Y'all can have two more in the NICU. Be quiet. Don't disturb other families."

Jeremiah held his grandmother's arm and escorted her to the side of Landon's crib. With a shaky hand, she caressed her great-grandson's head. Her knees buckled. Jeremiah and I grabbed her by the arms and held her. We then led her back to the waiting room.

After my time with Landon, I decided to make a quick trip to our home in the mountains. Not knowing how much longer we would be at the hospital, we needed a change of clothes and our toothbrushes. I wanted a shower, and I needed to get away from the pain at the hospital.

During the drive, I did not celebrate, as I did during the trip home on the previous day. Every song on the radio brought tears. After a shower at home, I changed clothes, packed a bag, grabbed my laptop computer, and headed back to the hospital in Winston-Salem. When I approached the city, a mid-afternoon rain shower passed through the area. Closer to the hospital, a giant rainbow appeared over the hospital. Maybe the God I read about in the Bible had sent a sign. The thought gave me comfort. I arrived back at the hospital a little before 5:00 p.m.

More friends and family arrived during my absence. I didn't want to talk. With a wireless Internet connection available, I wanted to get online and learn about my grandson's condition.

Malrotation with midgut volvulus, the medical term for what happened to Landon. What did it mean? What caused it?

In the corner of the waiting room, I read everything I could find. Landon, a worst-case scenario. His small intestine, dead. All of it. The information on the Internet confirmed the prognosis. The unfortunate occurrence sealed his fate - death. Nothing short of divine intervention could save him.

In the NICU, the pastor prayed for Landon again. Another family realized he was a preacher and asked him to pray for their child. Several minutes before he left, I saw him kneel with a different young mother in the waiting room, hold her hand, and pray for her sick baby.

By 8:00 p.m., the doctors completed their rounds. The pediatric surgeon stopped by the waiting room. No change. He would be back early the next morning for the second surgery.

The surgeon looked at me and motioned to follow him. In the hallway, the two of us walked together toward the elevator.

"You should make arrangements."

I knew what he meant.

The door to the elevator opened. The doctor stepped in.

I continued, past the elevator doors, to a quiet corner at the end of the hall. There, a large window revealed a nighttime view of the hospital entrance. I stood in front of the window, took a deep breath, and made a phone call to our hometown funeral director. I had known him most of my life. He handled the funerals for three of my grandparents and my father.

"Harold, I'm at Baptist Hospital. We've had a grandson born. He's not going to make it. I need to make arrangements for his funeral." My throat tightened. I paused to choke back a tear. "I need to come up with the money for the funeral. How much will it cost?"

"The funeral home will donate its services," Harold said. "My wife and I will buy a casket for the baby. The gravedigger won't charge anything."

I heard him say something, but the words didn't sink in. "How much will it cost?" I said.

"Eldon, I'm trying to tell you. If we don't have to transport the baby's body, it won't cost you anything. We don't charge to bury newborn babies. If your daughter-in-law is willing, when the baby dies, have the hospital wrap the body in a blanket and put him in his mother's arms. She can hold him while you drive them here. Bring the child's body straight to the funeral home."

"Thank you," I said. "I'll call you back when my grandson dies."

For several minutes, I stood in front of the window and stared into the black abyss.

I didn't want my family to know about the conversation with Harold. I arm wiped the tears from my cheeks, went to the cafeteria, got a cup of coffee, and sat alone at a table trying to compose myself.

When I returned to the waiting room, a little before 9:00 p.m., I discovered Jeremiah and Shelly sitting together, leaning forward, holding each other, crying.

"Oh, God, what's wrong? What happened?"

Kathy, standing in front of them, placed her hand on my arm. "A social worker asked them if they will donate Landon's organs for transplants. They said yes."

Of course, they will. Maybe something good could come

from Landon's short life.

However, I still couldn't understand why this happened. My grandson hadn't done anything to deserve this. My family hadn't done anything to deserve this. If there is a loving, compassionate God, why did he send this little child to us only to take him away so soon?

The pain, almost unbearable, made me angry. Where was God now?

Jeremiah's cell phone rang. He answered, and a puzzled expression crossed his face. He held the phone to his ear, stood, walked out of the waiting room, and down the hall.

Chapter 7

Transplant?

At 6:30 Wednesday morning, the sound of a metal cart banging against a door jolted me from a terrible dream. Awake, the reality was almost as bad.

Around me, Kathy, Roger, and Ezekiel slept in chairs on the left side of the room. Jeremiah slept in a chair in the corner; his wife curled beside him. Shelly moved, grabbed her abdomen, winced, then relaxed, and rested her head on Jeremiah's shoulder again.

I walked to a bathroom down the hall, leaned over a porcelain sink, and splashed cold water on my face. It soothed my swollen eyes. I rubbed the crusty matter at the corners and proceeded to brush my teeth, comb my hair, and return to the waiting room.

While my family still slept, I slipped into the NICU to see Landon. A squirt of hand sanitizer brought the smell of alcohol.

I braced.

The pediatric surgeon stood in the walkway a few feet from Landon's crib.

"Good day," I said.

The doctor, writing something on a chart, stopped and looked at me. "This is not going to be a good day. Unfortunately, for Landon, this will be a very bad day."

The look on his face revealed what he meant—Landon's last day.

"Are your son and daughter-in-law in the waiting room?"

My voice cracked, "They're asleep."

"In about an hour, we'll take Landon to the operating room."

Teary-eyed, I said, "I'll let them know."

"When we finish the surgery, I'll come to the waiting room to talk with your family."

I wiped the tears with the back of my hand, "Doctor, before you leave, a question. What should we expect? What will kill my grandson?"

The doctor, in his slow, methodical voice, said, "Landon's intestine will become septic. I'm surprised it hasn't happened by now. In Statesville, they gave him a powerful antibiotic, and we have continued to give it to him. The antibiotic has delayed infection. But soon, sepsis will take hold anyway and spread through Landon's body. His organs will shut down, and his heart will stop beating.

We will keep your grandson sedated. He will not suffer."

After the doctor left, I stood beside Landon's crib. Could this be his last day? I looked at my grandson. Did he know how much we loved him? Did he know we would be here with him until the end? I closed my eyes and became nauseous.

In the waiting room, I approached my son and gently touched his shoulder. He looked at me through one half-opened eye.

I whispered, trying not to wake Shelly, "They'll take Landon to surgery in about an hour. I'm hungry. I'm going to the cafeteria. I'll bring breakfast back for all of us."

He nodded and closed his eye.

In the cafeteria, I purchased six sausage biscuits, five small cartons of orange juice, and a coffee then returned to the waiting room.

Jeremiah slid away from his sleeping wife and placed his jacket under her head.

I offered him breakfast, but he needed the bathroom first.

While he was gone, I ate a biscuit and sipped hot coffee, which helped the queasiness in my stomach. Jeremiah returned, sat beside me, and unwrapped a biscuit. "Dad, last night, I talked to a woman. She told me something I need to talk to the doctor about."

Kathy and Shelly heard us talking and woke.

A few minutes later, the four of us stood and watched two nurses push Landon's crib toward the operating room.

I wrapped my arms around my wife and pulled her close. She laid her head on my shoulder and cried.

The second surgery didn't take long. The surgeon removed the tape, looked at the intestine, then replaced the tape. Afterward, the nurses brought Landon back to the NICU. Jeremiah and Shelly sat beside their son and waited for the surgeon to arrive with an update.

Kathy and I stayed in the waiting room with Roger and Ezekiel. We greeted friends and family when they arrived and helped them get into the NICU to see Landon. The woman – the gatekeeper at the counter – remained lenient. At first, we had four visitors with Landon. Then, with six visitors in the NICU, and being a little too loud, a nurse, polite and sympathetic, asked us to limit our visitors to four. The nurses, like us, expected today—day three—would be the last of Landon's short life.

About 11:00 a.m., the surgeon arrived in the hallway outside the waiting room. Two surgical nurses accompanied him—the three, dressed from head to toe in blue surgical scrubs. The surgeon instructed us to follow him to a conference room down the hall from the waiting room.

It wasn't big enough for all of us, so we stood close together. Several friends and family members were there, as well as the surgeon, the two surgical nurses, and a man dressed in a business suit.

Kathy nudged me and whispered, "That's the social worker who asked about donating Landon's organs."

In the conference room, we directed our attention toward the surgeon.

"Sorry to have taken so long to get here," he said. "We had emergency surgery after we finished with Landon. As for Landon, nothing has changed. His intestine is dead."

We expected this news. Still, we cried.

The doctor continued, "I can't say how long death will take. I'm sorry. I expect it will be soon."

A few visitors lowered their heads and sobbed.

Jeremiah spoke to the surgeon, "Doctor, last night, I got a phone call from a woman who works with Shelly." He looked at his wife, who stood beside him, then back at the doctor. "The woman told me her grandson was born, with his intestines twisted and on the outside of his body."

"Gastroschisis," the doctor said, "that's what you have described."

"She told me her grandson's intestine was dead, like Landon's. But her grandson didn't die. He received a small intestine and liver transplant at Georgetown University Hospital four years ago. He survived and is doing well." Jeremiah looked the doctor in the eye, "Is a transplant possible for Landon?"

The doctor stiffened and stepped back. He seemed to gather his thoughts before he said, "Intestinal transplants are relatively new and rare. Not many hospitals do them, none in North Carolina. They have not been very successful, especially with children." The doctor looked at the bewildered faces in the room and continued,

"Most children who have lived long enough to get a transplant have retained at least some of their small intestine. Landon has none. There are other factors to consider, and I'm not sure if he would be a candidate for a transplant."

Jeremiah, eyebrows raised, voice a little louder, spoke fast, inquiring, "How can we find out?"

"We'll need to contact a transplant surgeon at one of the hospitals doing intestinal transplants."

"The woman I spoke with last night gave me the numbers to the transplant surgeons at Georgetown."

One of the nurses, who stood beside the surgeon, excited, half-raised her hand and spoke, "Boston Children's Hospital does intestinal transplants. I worked on a transplant team in Boston. I'm sure the transplant doctor there would be happy to talk with you."

Jeremiah said, "Can we do that?"

"Yes," the surgeon nodded, "if you want me to, I'll call."

I said, "If there is any chance of my grandson surviving, we want to pursue it."

The doctor seemed relieved to end the meeting and eager to contact a transplant surgeon. His voice low, urgent, "If you and your family will return to the waiting room, I'll send someone to get you when we have a transplant doctor on the phone. Please don't get your hopes up." He made eye contact with Jeremiah and then with Shelly. "Even if Landon is a candidate for a transplant, he may not survive the next few hours, much less the months or years it would take for him to grow strong enough to survive a transplant. It's a long shot at best."

The surgeon, nurses, and social worker hurried out of the room to tend to Landon and research the possibility of a transplant.

Jeremiah and Shelly returned to the NICU. The rest of us headed to the waiting room.

Excited and confused, we discussed what happened. Intestinal transplant? I didn't know they could do that, was the common comment. They could. But could a transplant be possible for Landon? That was the question.

Around 3:00 p.m., the surgeon escorted Jeremiah and Shelly to a private room to talk with a transplant surgeon from Boston.

More visitors arrived and gathered with Kathy in the waiting room, where they talked about the conference call underway. A cousin murmured a quiet prayer.

Impatient, I paced and pondered—the woman whose grandson received an intestinal transplant, the nurse who had worked on a transplant team—how did they show up at the exact moment we needed them? The probabilities of coincidence seemed remote.

Had hours passed? I looked at my phone, 3:30. Only thirty minutes.

Finally, Jeremiah and Shelly entered the waiting room. We gathered around. Jeremiah looked at us and smiled. "We're going for a transplant."

A cheer erupted from our group.

"Yes, yes," I said, and repeated Jeremiah's words, "we're going for a transplant."

With my arms around my wife, I looked at her face. She smiled. Tears rolled down her cheeks.

I said, "Kathy, is it a dream?"

"No. You're not dreaming. Landon's got a chance."

We hugged our son and daughter-in-law.

Jeremiah said, "During the call, Landon's surgeon described, in detail, Landon's condition. The transplant surgeon explained to us what could go wrong and what might prevent Landon from getting a transplant. Yet, he told us if Landon survived the next few days, he believed Landon would be a good candidate for a transplant."

Again, cheers and smiles.

Jeremiah said, "We told Landon's surgeon we want to go for it. He agreed. He's scheduling another surgery to remove the dead intestine and to prepare Landon to survive until he gets a transplant. If he makes it through the surgery and the next few days, he's got a chance."

Jeremiah and Shelly returned to the NICU to sit with Landon.

We had hope.

Hope. A peculiar thing. It started small. The more we thought about it, the bigger it grew. Hope attracted other emotions—joy, happiness, love. Contagious, it spread from one person to another.

We hugged each other, laughed, and cried tears of joy.

Snatched from the depths of despair, we had hope.

Chapter 8

The Dead Intestine

Landon had a chance, but we still didn't know if he would survive. The dead intestine needed to come out before sepsis set in. We couldn't drop our guards. If Landon survived another surgery and days of recovery, maybe we could. Maybe.

About 5:00 p.m. Wednesday, two hours after the decision to go for a transplant, Jeremiah, who had been in the NICU with Shelly and Landon, came to the waiting room, where Kathy and I sat with visitors. He told us the surgeon had scheduled the third surgery for the next morning.

Livid, I stood and said, "Why can't the doctors do the surgery now? That dead intestine needs to come out."

"The surgeon said they couldn't get an operating room and couldn't get everything in place this late in the day."

I stomped my foot and raised my voice. "This is emergency surgery. I need to talk to the doctor."

"It's a complicated surgery." Jeremiah said, "We'll just have to wait until tomorrow."

Not wanting to upset my family by saying more, and annoyed that things were not happening the way I thought they should, I went to the cafeteria to cool off and gather my wits about me.

I drank a cup of coffee and thought about what Jeremiah said, "It's a complicated surgery." True. The surgeon would need all his resources and a plan in place to do a surgery to prepare Landon for his transplant journey. He couldn't rush. I returned to the waiting room, an hour later, in a better mood.

With the reprieve for Landon and the third surgery scheduled for the next day, most of the visitors left. Soon, only Jeremiah, Shelly, Roger, Ezekiel, Angie, Kathy, and I remained.

We didn't know how much longer we would be at the hospital; even if things went well, it could be weeks. Ezekiel had spent a night with Angie's family—away from the hospital. Roger had remained at the hospital near his sick brother for three days. The two previous nights, he slept in the waiting room. The boys needed to get away from the stressful, emotional situation, back to a normal routine and school.

A neighbor in Taylorsville offered to let Roger stay with them. Angie agreed to take him to the neighbor's house. She also offered to take Ezekiel home with her, again, for another night. Shelly smothered the boys with kisses, and about 6:30 p.m., Angie, Roger, and Ezekiel left.

Soon after, the social worker, who had been present at the morning meeting, joined us in the waiting room. Jeremiah, Shelly, Kathy, and I sat in the room eating sandwiches I had purchased at the hospital cafeteria.

"How are you holding up?" he said.

"We're tired, and we could use some good food," I said, holding a half-eaten sandwich for him to see.

He smiled, his eyes and voice compassionate. "There's a Ronald McDonald House across the street from the Hospital. Would you like me to put your family on the waiting list for a room?"

"Yes," Jeremiah said.

"Until then," he said, "I have arranged for you to get a family room here at the hospital. It's a private hospital room with a single bed, a private bathroom, and a shower. You can take turns using the room until one becomes available at the Ronald McDonald House."

He handed Jeremiah a small stack of paper tickets. "These are vouchers you can use to purchase food in the hospital cafeteria."

For a few seconds, the social worker didn't speak. The serious look on his face told me he struggled to find the right words. Finally, he found them. "Taking care of a child in need of a transplant is stressful. I've seen the stress tear families apart. You must learn how to provide specialized in-home medical care for your child, and you will need help. Can your family do this?"

"Yes," Jeremiah said, and he and Shelly nodded.

"My wife and I will help," I said. "We'll do whatever is necessary. I'm sure the rest of our family feels the same way."

"Okay," he said. "If there's anything I can do for you, please let me know. I'll let you know when a room becomes available at the Ronald McDonald House."

Wednesday evening, Jeremiah and Shelly went to the family room to sleep. Kathy and I stayed with Landon in the NICU. Often, during the night, I asked the nurse on duty about Landon's temperature; a rise could indicate sepsis. The nurse, likely tired of me asking, agreed to let me know if his temperature rose. Still, I couldn't relax. Sitting in a chair, beside his crib, I stared at my grandson and obsessed over the dead intestine.

His temperature remained the same.

Thursday morning, when Jeremiah and Shelly entered the NICU to relieve me of my watch, I placed my hand on Landon's forehead. Warm, but not hot. Reluctant yet tired, I left the NICU.

In the waiting room, exhausted and worried, Kathy and I waited for the surgery to begin. Sweat beaded on my forehead while I paced. I remembered the surgeon describing how the sepsis would kill Landon and looked at Kathy. "We're tempting fate, or God is watching over Landon. That intestine should have become septic by now. At least the surgery will start soon." It didn't.

9:00 a.m. came, and Landon remained in the NICU. At 10 a.m., a nurse told Jeremiah an emergency surgery had delayed Landon's surgery. Noon passed, and still, Landon had not left the

NICU.

Still, to this day, I wonder if something occurred behind the scenes—discussions or decisions we weren't aware of. Jeremiah and Shelly gave the okay to prepare Landon for a transplant, and the surgeon agreed. But, had the hospital agreed, the social workers, or Medicaid? Someone would have to pay for a transplant for Landon. We didn't have that kind of money.

With my anxiety level through the roof, I paced the hallways, answered phone calls, and replied to emails, all to keep my mind occupied. I needed to sleep but couldn't.

Kathy sat in the waiting room with her arms crossed on her chest, and her eyes closed. Yet, I could tell she wasn't asleep. She handled the stress by remaining motionless and praying. I paced.

That afternoon, still trying to stay calm and wanting to keep everyone informed about Landon's situation, I started a blog, called the Landon Joines Update Blog, landonjoines.blogspot.com. In 2009 we didn't use Facebook, Twitter, other social media sites, or even texts. We made phone calls and sent emails. I posted the first blog, and within a few minutes, dozens of people read the post. The blog gave me something to do, but soon anxiety about the dead intestine and sepsis returned. I paced the halls again.

Finally, at 4:20, I stood with Jeremiah, Shelly, and Kathy and watched the nurses push Landon's crib to the operating room. The four of us collapsed into chairs in the waiting room. With nothing to say, I tilted my head back and closed my eyes. I envisioned the surgeon removing the threat to my grandson's life. The anxiety left, and I relaxed enough to doze.

This surgery took longer than the first two.

In the operating room, careful to get all the necrotic tissue, the surgeon removed the dead intestine leaving about two centimeters or three-quarters of an inch of the small intestine at the bottom of Landon's duodenum. The surgeon connected the large intestine to the bottom of the duodenum. Technically, the duodenum is part of the small intestine. Landon might be able to absorb nutrition through his duodenum, but not much.

The surgeon placed a gastrostomy tube, or G-tube for short, through Landon's abdomen, into his stomach. Pumps would deliver formula, medicines, and fluids through the G-tube. Even though he didn't have a small intestine to absorb nutrition, his large intestine could absorb fluids.

The surgeon placed a temporary drain tube through the right side of Landon's abdomen, then stapled the incision closed. Next, he inserted a small white plastic tube, called a central line, through a vein in Landon's right thigh. He threaded the line through the vein and stopped with the end of the tube about an inch from Landon's heart. Pumps would force a nutritional formula, called total parenteral nutrition, or TPN, through the central line and into his bloodstream. With no other way to receive nourishment, Landon could not survive without the TPN. The surgeons finished the operation at 6:40 p.m., and a few minutes later, the nurses brought Landon back to the NICU, where we met them.

At 7:20 p.m., the surgeon came to the NICU. The surgery went well. The surgeon discovered a little inflammation, but no sign of sepsis. Still cautious, he ordered the nurses to continue administering antibiotics and watch for signs of infection. The effects of the sedative would wear off soon. Landon should begin to wake. The surgeon said, if Landon survived seventy-two hours with no major complications, he had a good chance.

Jeremiah, Shelly, Kathy, and I smiled and hugged each other. My son grasped the surgeon's hand and thanked him.

With the surgery finished, Jeremiah and I watched for signs of complications and of Landon waking. While we did, Shelly and Kathy returned to the birth Hospital, where a doctor removed the staples from Shelly's C-section incision and officially discharged her. Kathy and Shelly arrived back at Baptist hospital around 11:30, in time to witness Landon waking.

At 11:45 p.m., the sedation wore off, Landon moved his arms, and a few minutes later, for the first time since leaving the hospital in Statesville, three and a half days earlier, he opened his eyes.

Kathy used an expression that I often heard her mother and grandmother use, a long drawn out "Ooh," with rising pitch and an "ah," at the end. She has used it to express several things, amazement, admiration, love.

"Oohah, I see those beautiful blue eyes," Kathy said.

At 2:00 a.m. Friday, with the dead intestine removed and the third surgery over, we felt good about Landon's condition. I smiled at my wife, looked into her eyes, and said, "Let's go home."

Kathy drove. I slept. At home, in our bed, we slept a few more hours.

Friday morning, we ate a good breakfast, took a shower,

changed clothes, checked on my mother, and arrived back at the hospital about lunchtime.

Jeremiah met us in the waiting room with good news. Landon's hemoglobin increased to an acceptable level, the nurses hadn't detected any signs of infection, and the Ronald McDonald House granted Jeremiah and Shelly a room. Even better, Kathy and I could use it.

Friday afternoon, my son and daughter-in-law walked to the Ronald McDonald House. A volunteer gave them a tour and briefed them on the policies. Kathy and I stayed with Landon.

Twenty-four hours after the third surgery, we sat in chairs beside of our grandson's crib, watched the monitors, and listened to the slow, steady beep they made.

Landon slept while the ventilator swooshed and pumped oxygen into his lungs.

After a few minutes, he opened his eyes. I sat on the edge of my chair and watched. He thrashed his arms, moved his head from side to side, and fought against the ventilator. A nurse came in and increased the flow of his pain medication to help him relax. Kathy stood beside his crib. She caressed his head. Soon, Landon stopped struggling, closed his eyes, and slept again. I slid back in my chair and relaxed.

Fifteen minutes later, a sudden, rapid, beeping of an alarm startled me. I jumped from the chair. Landon's heart rate slowed, and fell below the alarm threshold.

The nurse rushed in, turned off the alarm, made some

adjustments, turned to me, and said, "Too much pain medication." She looked at the monitors. "He's okay."

I returned to my chair and placed my hand on my throat. The drumbeat in my ears kept time with my pounding heart until my heart rate returned to normal.

A few minutes later, Kathy held Landon's hand while I caressed his forehead with my fingertips. I looked at his little face and sensed his strong will to live.

Kathy leaned over his crib and whispered, "Come on, little guy. You can make it."

Her watery eyes revealed her love for our grandson.

A few minutes later, our son and daughter-in-law returned from the Ronald McDonald House. Jeremiah went to Taylorsville to pick up his two oldest sons and take them home.

Shelly, Kathy, and I had decided I would take a short nap then return to the hospital to stay with Landon during the night.

That evening, while the sun disappeared behind the Blue Ridge, I walked to the Ronald McDonald House.

Spring had arrived. Winston-Salem bloomed. Tulips, daffodils, dogwoods, and azaleas filled the yards and lined the sidewalks. Sweet smells floated on warm breezes. Within a few minutes, I stood in front of the house. In the yard, flowers and shrubs bloomed along a manicured brick walkway leading to the front door.

During their orientation, a volunteer gave Jeremiah and Shelly a code to enter the house. I used it. Inside, a volunteer greeted me and gave me a quick tour.

Large seating areas with sofas, televisions, and desks provided a cozy place to get away from the stresses at the hospital.

In the kitchen, well-stocked refrigerators and cabinets contained free food for the guest.

Several nights each week, local volunteers, church groups, or civic organizations brought or prepared free meals.

The volunteer took me to our room.

The bedroom, small, quiet, with a double bed and a private bathroom, would serve us well.

I stretched out on the bed and reflected on the events of the past four days. People had arrived, and things had happened that I didn't understand—the doctors, the pastor, the grandmother, the nurse, and the dead intestine that remained in Landon's abdomen for almost four days without becoming septic.

What I previously believed about God changed. Convinced these events couldn't have happened by chance, God placed these people in the right place at the right time; He had taken care of Landon. I said a prayer for my grandson, then slept.

Chapter 9

After Surgery
and The Advocate

Landon continued to recover from the third surgery, and our family continued to recover from the shock of the events surrounding his birth. There were setbacks, scares, and unexpected problems. But with each passing hour, his condition improved, and we adjusted to the new normal.

Friday evening, I returned to the NICU for the overnight shift. Kathy and Shelly went to the Ronald McDonald House to sleep.

I sat in a chair and watched for signs of healing or, heaven forbid, signs of something wrong. A few times, Landon's heart rate fluctuated, or his blood pressure changed, both attributed to the pain medication.

Each time this happened, the nurse checked Landon, looked at me, smiled, and said, "He's okay."

Saturday, about 2:00 a.m., the nurse hung a bag of TPN on a pole. She connected a tube from the bag to Landon's central line.

A few years earlier, TPN didn't exist. Without it, he would not survive. I stared at the bag of life-sustaining formula and then at Landon's snow-white face. His face reminded me of a song I sang to my other grandsons when they were infants. In a low, whispered voice, I sang about how God sent His love on the wings of a snow-white dove. I sang slow, the way Robert Duvall did in the movie *Tender Mercies*.

I sensed God's love for my grandson, flowing through me. I witnessed a miracle, not in the form of a dove, but in the life of this fragile baby. I continued to hum the tune while hours passed. The night turned to morning.

Saturday morning, Jeremiah, Roger, and Ezekiel returned to Winston-Salem. They didn't come to the NICU but went to the Ronald McDonald House to see Shelly and Kathy. Together, the five walked to the hospital.

Kathy and I took Roger and Ezekiel home for the remainder of the weekend.

The boys fished in the trout stream behind our house, and Roger reeled in a nice twelve-inch brown trout. For a brief time, away from the hospital, they laughed and enjoyed themselves.

Jeremiah and Shelly promised to call if anything went wrong with Landon. It didn't. He continued to recover.

Sunday afternoon, eager to visit Landon, we returned to the hospital. We walked into the NICU and found him less sedated, more alert, and breathing without the ventilator. With his eyes wide open, he looked at us, mostly at Kathy. A tube still ran through his nose to his stomach. Another tube supplied oxygen. A strip of white tape, under his nose and across his face, held the tubes in place. With the ventilator removed and less swelling in his face, to us, he looked good.

Sunday evening, seventy-two hours after the third surgery, a milestone set by the surgeon, Landon, almost a week old, continued to recover. We smiled, hugged each other, and relaxed a little bit more.

To celebrate and spend time with their older sons, Jeremiah and Shelly took Roger and Ezekiel out for a meal at a nearby restaurant.

Kathy and I stayed at the hospital and took turns in the NICU with Landon. When not with our grandson, we greeted visitors in the waiting room. Many told us their churches prayed for Landon earlier that morning.

His story touched people. Several told us how they felt a nudge from God to call or come to the hospital to pray for Landon. We prayed with them. We told them about Landon's progress and how happy it made us, but also spoke about the long journey ahead and asked if they would continue to pray for him. All agreed. Soon, hundreds, if not thousands, would be praying for Landon.

Jeremiah and Shelly returned to the hospital in time to meet with some of the visitors.

The steady stream of phone calls and visits from well-wishers lifted our spirits, yet at the same time, it exhausted us. Recovering from one of the most traumatic weeks of our lives, we needed a sense of normalcy and a return to a routine.

Late Sunday evening, Shelly and the boys went home, Kathy and I left, while Jeremiah stayed with Landon.

The manager of the restaurant where Shelly worked scheduled her to return to work on Saturday, five days after giving birth by C-section, because of Landon's situation, she didn't. She called the restaurant on Friday, explained why she couldn't work, and promised to either call again or return to work on Monday.

Monday, Shelly got her two older sons to school and then drove to a gas station where she used her last twelve dollars on gas for the Lincoln. The big, comfortable car guzzled gas. Twelve dollars would buy her enough to get to work and back for two days. With the family low on funds, she needed to work.

When Shelly arrived at the restaurant, the manager fired her. He cited subpar performance on the last day she worked, hours before giving birth, and not working Saturday and Sunday, as reasons for her dismissal.

Shelly couldn't believe what happened. With watery eyes, she, once again, told about Landon and why she didn't work when scheduled. She begged for her job because her family needed the money. But the manager wouldn't listen. Her disbelief turned to anger, and she raised her voice in protest. The manager threatened to call the police if Shelly didn't leave quietly. She did, in tears.

In the parking lot, she called Jeremiah to tell him what

happened. Jeremiah told her to go home, get some rest, and forget about the job. Somehow, they would make ends meet.

Kathy and I owned a small upholstery shop where the two of us worked. Monday, we opened our business for the first time in more than a week. We toiled but couldn't focus. We thought about our grandson, still in the NICU.

Our shop phone rang.

Jeremiah spewed out the words, "Dad, Shelly lost her job. We don't have any money. I don't have any jobs finished, so I can't collect any money. Shelly doesn't even have enough gas to get back to the hospital. I don't know what to do."

"Son, calm down. I'm sorry about Shelly's job, but don't worry about it. The two of you concentrate on Landon. Your mom and I will help. We have a couple of jobs we can finish today and get paid for tomorrow. We'll take Shelly some money."

After the phone call, nauseated, I lowered my face into my hands. Our business supported Kathy and me, but I didn't know how much we could help Jeremiah and his family. I knew, though, somehow, we would. Our work took on new importance.

We didn't know it at the time, but God blessed Shelly by taking her job away. He gave her a new full-time job, caring for Landon. It didn't pay anything, but Shelly became an excellent caregiver. God knew what needed to happen.

At the hospital, the nurses continued to wean Landon from the pain medication. Monday afternoon, they removed the tube, which went through his nose, to his stomach. They also removed the oxygen tube and the tape from his face. Jeremiah emailed us pictures.

"Oohah, he looks good," Kathy said

Monday night, Jeremiah went to the Ronald McDonald House to sleep. He left Landon in the care of the nurses.

About 2:00 a.m., a nurse called him and said, "Something's wrong with Landon, come to the NICU."

He ran to the hospital. There, a nurse told him Landon developed supraventricular tachycardia, a dangerous, fast heart rate. Probably a result of withdrawing from the pain medication. The nurses placed ice packs around Landon's neck and hoped the cold would slow his heart rate. It did. Within a few minutes, his racing heart slowed and returned to normal.

Terrified by the episode, Jeremiah refused to leave Landon for more than a few minutes. Our family realized that we couldn't leave Landon's care in the hands of anyone. It's not that we couldn't; we didn't want to. And, it's not that anyone did anything wrong. We saw how quickly things could go bad, and we wanted to be there for Landon if it did again.

After the scare at the hospital, I thought about what the future held for Landon and my family. I wondered what our roles would be in caring for him and getting him a transplant.

Jeremiah and Shelly would have their hands full with his day-to-day care, Kathy would help with Roger and Ezekiel, and I would work and help with the finances. We would support our family. But what else could I do?

People who know me will tell you I am a take-charge person. I can't help it. I need to know everything about a situation, and if I can control it, I will. Sometimes when I can't, I still try until I realize I shouldn't.

The way we found out about a transplant led me to believe we couldn't depend on the doctors to give us all the information we needed to make decisions about Landon's care. The doctors didn't withhold information from us. They followed the protocol of the time for children in Landon's situation. But recent progress in intestinal transplants made it possible for children like Landon to receive one, and the protocol hadn't changed to keep up with the advancements. When we discovered Landon could be a candidate for a transplant, it shocked the doctors as much as it did us. For us to help Landon, we needed to learn more about intestinal transplants. We couldn't expect doctors to know everything, and I remembered the pain I felt when the surgeon told us Landon was going to die. We couldn't leave decisions concerning Landon's care in the hands of doctors or anyone else.

I would become Landon's advocate.

In 2009 not many businesses in our little hometown had Internet service. Although recently installed, we did. Several times, while I worked, something would come to my mind. I paused my work, ran to my computer, and search for information. I read everything I could find—web pages, medical journals, articles, and blogs. I printed pages of information, highlighted lines, wrote notes in margins. I prepared so I could tell the doctors what needed to happen, not the other way around.

Two days of research left me with a notebook full of questions about Landon and what we should do for him. I needed answers. Landon's surgeon would be an excellent place to start.

6:00 a.m. Wednesday, prepared to intercept the surgeon during morning rounds, I left home in my Ford pickup truck and drove to the hospital.

I arrived at the NICU to find the nurses excited. Landon pooped! That's right, ten days after his birth, he made his first messy diaper. The nurses had pumped formula through the G-tube and into his stomach, and it came out the other end. The plumbing worked, another milestone on the recovery road.

"Way to go, Landon," a nurse said while she changed his diaper.

A few minutes later, Landon's surgeon arrived at the NICU. The doctor, gracious, answered as many questions as he could. Then he said we need to schedule a family meeting. He agreed to arrange a meeting with representatives from all departments involved with Landon's care. They could answer my questions and help us develop a plan. I wanted to talk with the different departments, informed and on their level, as best I could. To do that, I needed even more information and continued to dig.

Wednesday afternoon, seeking more answers, I made a phone call to the transplant doctor in Boston, the same doctor Jeremiah and Shelly talked to a week earlier.

The doctor, already familiar with Landon's case, told me what needed to happen for Landon to get a transplant and the things that could go wrong. He said Landon faced many threats that could kill him. One of the biggest would be liver failure.

Infants must have lipids—fats—in their nutrition to aid in organ development and function. Pharmaceutical companies derive the lipids used in the TPN administered to Landon, from vegetable oils or soybean oil. These fats gunk up the liver and lead to liver failure, especially in children. Not all infants on long-term TPN develop liver failure. In those that do, it can happen quickly, resulting in the need for both a liver and small intestine transplant. That's what happened to the grandson of the woman who worked with Shelly.

Earlier, I read the blogs of several children with medical conditions like Landon's. Most of those children who received long-term TPN developed liver damage. Several received multi-visceral transplants. Their stories touched my heart. A few of the children had died either of liver failure before they could get a transplant or of complications afterward. Reading their stories made me even more aware of Landon's uncertain future.

The transplant doctor told me about the Center for Advanced Intestinal Rehabilitation (CAIR) at Boston Children's Hospital and how they specialized in caring for Short Bowel Syndrome (SBS) children, like Landon.

A research project underway at Boston Children's Hospital showed promising results in saving the livers of children on TPN, using a lipid called Omegaven. Researchers in Germany developed this lipid from fish oil instead of vegetable oil. In some children, this new lipid formula stopped the liver damage, and in a few cases, reversed it.

The doctor in Boston said if the level of Landon's liver enzymes—bilirubin—rose, that could be an indicator of liver damage, and it would be imperative we get Landon on Omegaven as soon as possible.

There might be a problem, Omegaven did not have FDA approval, and Landon couldn't receive it except on a humanitarian basis. The thought of this infuriated me. The FDA wouldn't let Landon have this liver saving formula until after his liver failed and death was imminent. It didn't make sense to me.

Our other option would be to get him enrolled in the research project in Boston. But how?

Every answer led to more questions. For me to protect my grandson, be his advocate, and help him get a transplant, I needed to learn much more.

Wednesday evening, Landon's surgeon informed us that the hospital had scheduled the family meeting for Friday at 10:00 a.m.

When Jeremiah called to tell Shelly about the family meeting, she was crying. She hadn't seen her son in almost three days. She wanted to come to the hospital but had no money. Kathy drove to Taylorsville, gave Shelly cash for gas, and then stayed with Roger and Ezekiel.

At the hospital, it didn't take Jeremiah and Shelly long to discover another problem, diaper rash.

The formula pumped through Landon's G-tube and into his stomach mixed with digestive juices, and soon ended up in his diaper. Acidic. Caustic. It burned his bottom. Within a few diaper changes, his butt turned red. After a few more, it blistered, and the skin peeled.

Jeremiah, Shelly, and the nurses experimented with different gels, creams, and powders. They looked for something that would protect Landon's bottom. Nothing worked. Keeping his bottom dry, with frequent diaper changes, helped.

Thursday evening, I sat at our dining room table with my laptop computer and prepared for the meeting at the hospital the next day. I stayed up late and researched. I studied as if preparing for a final exam, except this was much more important. The research and the conversations with Landon's surgeon and the transplant doctor answered a lot of my questions. But they also revealed many ways things could go wrong, keep Landon from getting a transplant, and kill him. We needed a plan to prevent those things from happening and a plan leading to a transplant. I hoped the family meeting would help us make such a plan.

Late in the evening, I fell asleep with my head on the table in front of my computer.

Chapter 10

Nurse Training and The Family Meeting

Prepared for the meeting, I arrived at the hospital at about 9:00 a.m. Friday, May 1, 2009—eleven days after Landon's birth. I wanted more information about how to get Landon a transplant. Jeremiah and Shelly, tired of living in the hospital, wanted to know how to get Landon home.

I met my son and daughter-in-law in the NICU and visited with Landon for a few minutes before the meeting scheduled for 10:00 a.m. His face showed no sign of pain or distress while he thrashed his arms and cooed. The yellow onesie outfit and the rosy color of his cheeks made him look healthy. My day became brighter when I saw him active and happy.

I stood beside the crib, gazed at my grandson, and thought about how blessed we were to still have him with us. A scheduled diaper change interrupted the doting.

Shelly wiped his raw bottom, and he squirmed and cried. His cries sent cold chills down my back. Shelly coated his bottom with white ointment, sprinkled powder on it, and placed a new diaper on his bottom.

She leaned over Landon's crib and placed her face close to his. "I'm sorry," she whispered.

A few minutes later, the diaper change over, Landon again cooed and moved his arms as if nothing had happened. I didn't change many diapers. Kathy did. And, I cringed each time I heard Landon cry.

Kathy, who stayed the night before with Roger and Ezekiel at their home, got them off to school, then drove to the hospital. She arrived about fifteen minutes before the meeting and sat with Landon while Jeremiah, Shelly, and I met the doctors, nurses, and hospital staff.

A large rectangle table filled the conference room. We sat at one end. At the other, the head nurse and two nurses from the NICU talked. On the left sat a representative from the pharmacy and another from the financial department. The social worker and the surgeon sat on the right.

The length of the table made us feel distant from the nurses at the other end, yet we could hear the conversation.

The head nurse held a lab report and discussed Landon's TPN formula with the pharmacist. The nurse pointed at the paper. They talked about what nutrients and vitamins to mix in the TPN and how much of each.

Even though the TPN supplied his nutrition, he still needed formula pumped into his stomach through the G-tube so his stomach and large intestine would remain active. The nurses said they had stopped the G-tube feedings because Landon vomited when fluids entered his stomach. The vomiting could cause Landon to aspirate or suck fluids into his lungs, which could lead to pneumonia.

The head nurse suggested the nurses try to restart the feeds with small amounts of formula.

Shelly said, "An increase in the G-tube feeds will increase the output in his diaper. He already has a terrible diaper rash. What can we do?"

I shuddered at the thought of more diaper changes for Landon.

The pharmacist suggested a cream that might be helpful. She would send a tube to the NICU for Landon.

Jeremiah leaned forward and looked at the surgeon. "When can we take our baby home?"

The doctor said, "Who will be his primary caregiver?"

"We will," said Jeremiah and Shelly, in unison.

"Both of you need to learn how to change his TPN bags, control the pumps, connect formula for G-tube feedings, administer medicines, and keep everything sterile." He pointed at the nurses at the end of the table. "You'll need to shadow these nurses. Learn what they do. When I'm convinced you can take care of your son at home, I'll discharge him."

Jeremiah placed his hand on Shelly's. "We can do this."

I smiled and beamed with pride at the confidence in my son's voice.

The surgeon said, "You will need to establish a sterile area in your home to do line changes and handle the central line."

I thought of the small home and wondered where my son and daughter-in-law would find a space to keep sterile.

Shelly, focused on getting Landon home, asked a logistical question. "How will we get the TPN for Landon when we get home?"

The pharmacist said, "We'll mix the TPN here at the hospital, pack it in coolers with medicines and supplies, and a courier will deliver to your home each week."

The social worker looked at both parents and said, "You'll have help at home. A nurse will visit, not every day, but often."

Having done the research, I already knew the answer to this question. Still, I wanted to hear what the surgeon had to say. "What can kill Landon?"

Without hesitation, he said, "A line infection."

A line infection happens when bacteria enters the central line and then the bloodstream. The bacteria can infect the organs, cause septic shock and death. A fever is the first sign of a line infection.

The surgeon said, "If he gets a fever, get him back to the hospital fast. We'll treat him with antibiotics and might need to remove the infected central line. Most often, scarring prevents us from using the site again."

"Can you place the line somewhere else?" I said.

"Yes, but with only six access sites on the body, one in each thigh, each side of the chest, and each side of the neck, it's possible to run out of sites."

Jeremiah said, "What happens if he runs out of access sites?"

The surgeon interlocked his fingers, placed his arms on the table, and looked at Jeremiah, "Your son will have no way to get nutrition. He'll die. You must protect these precious sites."

Six access sites sounded like plenty. It wasn't.

I looked at the surgeon and said, "What else can kill him?"

"Liver failure," he said.

"I've read about how the lipids in the TPN cause liver failure," I said. "Omegaven has helped other children. Can we get it for Landon?"

The surgeon shook his head. "Without FDA approval, I don't think you'll ever get Omegaven for Landon in North Carolina. If his liver goes bad, he'll receive a liver transplant as well as an intestinal transplant."

I shook my head. We wouldn't allow the TPN to damage Landon's liver without a fight.

I said, "The research I have done shows the dismal mortality rates of children who have received a liver and intestinal transplant. Liver failure made the children sick, too sick to survive a transplant.

He needs Omegaven."

The surgeon said, "We want to prevent the lipids from damaging Landon's liver also, but as I said, Omegaven is not an option for us."

I leaned forward and made eye contact with the surgeon. "It is in Boston."

He pursed his lips then looked away from me. Had I said something wrong or hurtful?

I didn't mean to, but the solution seemed simple. If the vegetable oil-based lipids damaged Landon's liver, give him the fish oil-based Omegaven. Yet, with the FDA and Medicaid involved, it wasn't simple. The FDA blocked Omegaven, and Medicaid held the purse strings.

The hospital staff knew we were not a wealthy family.

"Medicaid will cover most of your son's medical expenses," the financial representative said. "Yet it won't pay for things like travel, lodging, and supplies. We've seen these expenses become an overwhelming burden for some families."

The tone was compassionate, yet to me, it sounded like the words meant for low-income families, like ours.

The surgeon said, "When the time comes for Landon's transplant, the surgery will happen at a hospital a long distance from here. You'll need to stay near the hospital for many months, maybe a year. Other families have done fundraisers to help with these expenses."

My ears perked. Through my involvement with Scouts, other non-profit organizations, and charities, I knew how to raise money. "We could do a fundraiser for my grandson."

The financial woman said, "You must be careful in how you raise money for Landon. Any funds donated must be counted as income and could impact Landon's eligibility for Medicaid."

"How can we raise the money we need?" I said.

The social worker said, "You'll need to get a lawyer to establish a trust. It's complicated and difficult to administer. Or, you could go through a non-profit organization whose purpose is to help with situations like yours. I'm sure you could find one on the Internet."

More research. Something I could do.

The medical team at Baptist Hospital answered most of our questions. After the meeting, Jeremiah and Shelly focused on getting out of the hospital and taking their son home. I focused on preparing the way for Landon to get a transplant.

In the first two weeks of Landon's life, I witnessed God perform a miracle. Still, I didn't have enough faith to believe He would protect my grandson and keep him alive—without my help. He needed me. But I feared if I missed one little detail, Landon would die, and it would be my fault.

I couldn't let that happen.

Chapter 11

Liver Damage and The Homecoming

Bringing a newborn home is exciting, and with Landon, even more so. When the surgeon told us Landon would not leave the hospital alive, we gave up hope of him ever coming home. By the grace of God, if everything went as planned, he would soon, very much alive.

After the family meeting, the nurses moved Landon out of the NICU and to an intermediate care ward. There, under the guidance and watchful eyes of the nurses, Jeremiah and Shelly learned the nursing skills needed to care for their son.

The numerous instructions the nurses gave overwhelmed Jeremiah and Shelly. They couldn't remember everything, and one mistake could cost Landon his life. Jeremiah bought a notebook where he recorded as much as he could. He made schedules, noted medicines and dosages. He wrote detailed instructions on how to manage the pumps and how to keep everything sterile. Shelly, in addition to the usual care and cuddling a mother gives a newborn, learned to administer medicines, connect G-tube lines, and control the pumps. Both parents watched to ensure a line didn't become tangled, snagged, or get jerked. Accidentally jerking the central line out could cause Landon to bleed to death in a matter of minutes.

A few times, the long hours, constant watching, and stress in the hospital caused exhaustion. As Jeremiah recalls, they took turns going to the Ronald McDonald House and collapsing on the bed.

Jeremiah and Shelly focused on Landon. Although the older sons seemed to take the situation in stride, they needed attention also. For two nights, they stayed with Angie. Then Kathy went to the family home and cared for them there. She got them to school, prepared their meals, and tried to create an atmosphere of normalcy.

Roger, quiet, stayed in his bedroom and played his guitar.

Several times Ezekiel asked, "Is my little brother still going to die?"

Kathy choked back tears and did her best to comfort Ezekiel.

Everything went well until Wednesday, May 6, five days after the family meeting, when Landon's bloodwork revealed high bilirubin levels. The test indicated the lipid in the TPN might have already damaged his liver. I didn't think this would happen so soon. My research showed if Landon's bilirubin remained high, he could be in liver failure within three months. Had God saved him from sepsis at birth, only to have him die of liver failure a few months later?

Alarmed, Landon's surgeon and Jeremiah had an urgent conference call with the transplant doctor in Boston. They agreed to reduce the lipids and prescribed Landon a drug called Actigall. The drug is used to dissolve gall stones and is also used to treat liver disease. Because of side effects, the drug can't be used for long but might help as a quick short-term fix. Concerned about the rise in the bilirubin, yet hopeful it wouldn't delay the plan to bring Landon home, we continued with the preparations.

On Saturday, May 9, a week after last seeing their parents and brother, Kathy and I took Roger and Ezekiel to the hospital for a visit. In the elevator, Roger, in a rare talkative, almost giddy mood, said, "I can't wait 'till Landon gets to come home, and our family can be together." In the hall, near Landon's room, Ezekiel ran ahead of us.

When we entered the room, Jeremiah wrapped his arms around Ezekiel's shoulders and announced, "Landon gained weight this week. The doctor said if the hospital can get everything in order, we can take him home next week."

Roger let out a "Woohoo." I hugged Jeremiah, then my wife.

She looked at her grandson in his crib. "Can you believe it, Landon, you get to go home?"

He smiled as if he understood.

He also smiled when he saw his brothers, then thrashed his arms and kicked his legs. Both older boys laughed and tickled their little brother under his chin. The three played for several minutes before the smell indicated one of them needed a diaper change.

Landon cried and squirmed while Kathy cleaned his bottom.

"His butt's not as red."

Jeremiah handed his mother a tube of cream. "The pharmacy sent this. It seems to help."

After she changed the diaper, Kathy whispered to Landon, "I'm sorry."

He whimpered, then drank a little formula from a bottle.

Jeremiah, eager to demonstrate his new skills, said, "Landon needs a line change. We've waited until you got here to do it so we could show you how." Roger, Ezekiel, Kathy, and I watched from across the room—far enough away that we wouldn't contaminate anything. Jeremiah and Shelly put on yellow paper gowns, hair nets, masks, and latex gloves. With focused and intense movements, Jeremiah followed the instructions written in his notebook. A nurse watched the parents work together and complete the complicated procedure. When they finished, she said, "Well done."

The dressing on Landon's thigh around the central line access site needed changing as well.

Shelly removed the tape and gauze. "Oh my gosh, look how red it is," she said and called the nurse over to look.

While they talked, Kathy and I eased close enough to see. I noticed that the redness on Landon's thigh was the same shape as the tape Shelly had removed. We didn't know it at the time, but this allergy would become a significant problem. Shelly and the nurse decided to clean the site, place new gauze around the line, and recheck it at the next cleaning.

I marveled at how much my son and daughter-in-law learned in such a short time.

Roger, Ezekiel, Kathy, and I had something to learn too. That afternoon we took a CPR class.

Afterward, Kathy and I took Roger and Ezekiel to our home for another weekend of fishing.

Shelly went home to clean the house and make final preparations in the hope that Landon could come home soon. She didn't just clean the house; she did her best to sterilize it. Jeremiah stayed at the hospital. With the help of the nurses, he tended to Landon.

The hospital staff worked several days trying to locate a home health nurse for Landon. Most of the home health providers that served the rural area where the family lived didn't have a nurse qualified to care for an infant with a central line and as fragile as Landon. The doctor wouldn't let Landon go home if the hospital couldn't locate and hire one. Finally, after numerous phone calls, the hospital staff found a qualified nurse about 25 miles from the family home. She agreed to take the assignment. She would meet the family when Landon arrived home, clearing the way for Landon's homecoming.

Sunday evening, our home phone rang. I exchanged greetings with Jeremiah before he said, "If nothing bad happens, we can take Landon home tomorrow."

I smiled and gave Kathy a silent thumbs-up. She knew what I meant. Through teary eyes, she smiled back.

"We'll be there," I said.

At 5:00 a.m. Monday morning, eager to get the day started, I jumped out of bed. I had work to do before Kathy and I could put a "Closed" sign on our business door and head to the family home to welcome Landon.

After they got their boys off to school, Angie drove Shelly to the hospital, where the two helped Jeremiah pack Landon's things, receive final instructions from the doctor, and sign the discharge papers.

I expected Jeremiah and Shelly to grab Landon and exit the hospital as fast as they could. They didn't. They had become attached to the nurses who treated Landon. For several minutes they exchanged hugs and tears. A few of those nurses still follow Landon's story.

That afternoon, three weeks after Landon's birth, Kathy and I drove to Taylorsville. On the way, we purchased six blue helium-filled balloons from a Walmart. At the home, Kathy and Ezekiel tied the balloons to the rails around the front porch. Ezekiel, restless, punched the balloons while we waited.

The home nurse got lost on the country roads but arrived a few minutes before Landon. After introductions, Kathy, Roger, and I stood on the porch and talked with the nurse.

It might have been nerves, but the nurse's voice quivered when she spoke. Trying to ease the tension with a conversation, I asked if she had ever tended to a child with a central line. She said yes, with an older child, but not with an infant. I sensed a lack of confidence. Was she the right nurse for Landon?

In the yard, Ezekiel jumped and shouted, "Here they come."

We rushed to the driveway. Angie arrived first with Shelly and Landon in the back seat of her blue sedan. Jeremiah followed. Milo, the big black Lab mixed family dog, wagged his tail and ran beside both vehicles.

Ezekiel opened his mother's door. Kathy and I leaned forward and peered over Shelly at Landon in his car seat.

Shelly stepped out of the car, turned her back to us, then careful not to snag the tubes, pulled the infant carrier from the vehicle. She turned and presented Landon to our family.

Kathy said, "Oohah, there he is. Hey, sweetie."

I wrapped an arm around my wife's shoulder. Through tear-filled eyes, we marveled at the little boy squinting in the bright daylight.

Ezekiel touched Landon's cheek. Roger stood behind Ezekiel, looked at his youngest brother in the carrier, and smiled.

Shelly said, "Let me get him in the house. It's cold out here." She tucked the blanket in the carrier around Landon's shoulders and headed for the door, stopping to show Landon the balloons before entering.

Shelly sat the carrier on the sofa. Kathy unbuckled Landon, pulled him from the seat, held him close, and rocked from side to side.

Jeremiah and I carried boxes of medical supplies and a cooler full of bags of TPN into the house. Jeremiah loaded the TPN, which must remain cold, in the new dorm size refrigerator his wife purchased the day before and placed on their bedroom floor. Shelly and the home nurse unpacked the boxes. They stored the supplies in a kitchen cabinet Shelly had cleaned out, for that purpose. They talked about and made notes of where they placed everything.

With the TPN and supplies put away, I sat in a chair in the living room, watched Kathy hold Landon, and listened while Jeremiah and Shelly talked with the nurse, who no longer showed signs of nervousness. The three discussed the TPN, the pumps, and medicines. Jeremiah showed the nurse his notebook full of notes about Landon's care. They also talked about the nurse's schedule and responsibilities. The doctor ordered her to come every other day, record Landon's weight, vital signs, and test his blood sugar. Each week she would draw blood for a blood test.

The nurse said she would do the line changes. Jeremiah and Shelly said they could and insisted they would. She agreed without an argument.

An hour later, with the schedule decided, the nurse left. A wave of fear came over me when I realized there were no medical professionals there to tend to Landon—just us. I had confidence in my son and daughter-in-law. They knew what to do, but I felt the weight of the responsibility also.

A few minutes later, hamburgers sizzled on a grill. The smell drifted through the little house. Shelly sliced tomatoes and peeled leaves of lettuce.

Outside, Ezekiel rode his four-wheeler around the property. He cruised slowly while he gazed through the forest and across the meadows, as if deep in thought, or content.

Back in the house, Roger played a beautiful rendition of Pink Floyd's, "Wish You Were Here," on an acoustic guitar. He practiced the song a lot while his brother and parents were away. Kathy hummed along.

Landon fell asleep in his grandmother's arms. She carried him to the bedroom. I followed close behind, held the small black bag with the pumps inside, and kept the lines from getting snagged. Kathy laid him in his new crib. I hung the pumps and bags of TPN on a pole beside the crib while Kathy covered him with the little blue blanket. We held each other and gazed at our grandson.

"He looks peaceful," Kathy said. "Can you believe he's home?"

Jeremiah, who tended the grill in the back yard, shouted, "The hamburgers are ready."

With the family together, at home, for the first time in weeks, everything seemed right.

After he wolfed down a burger, Jeremiah sat sideways on the sofa with one leg on a cushion, the other on the floor. He leaned back, rested his head on his arm, and closed his eyes. I looked at his pale face. He yawned. I thought about the previous three weeks and what my thirty-three-year-old son had endured. Hours without sleep, extreme emotional swings, and back pain didn't get him down. He held strong. During those three weeks, I don't think he slept a deep sleep.

Now, on his sofa, with his son home, he did.

Chapter 12

The Battle with Medicaid

We loved having Landon at home. Life got a little easier. But a few days later, the first signs of trouble appeared, and within a month, we were in a fight with Medicaid.

Medicaid allows a bureaucrat to decide who gets the best treatment and who doesn't, not the doctors or the family. At least that's what almost happened to Landon.

Nine days after coming home, Jeremiah, Shelly, and Landon made the 100-mile roundtrip from the family home to the surgeon's office for a scheduled visit. The surgeon handed Jeremiah a paper with the results of Landon's weekly bloodwork.

Jeremiah looked at the paper and shook his head. "What happened?"

Concern was written all over the surgeon's face. "The Actigall worked and kept his liver enzymes down for a brief time, but the bilirubin is rising again. Other than monitoring the test results, there's not much we can do."

Jeremiah instructed the surgeon to fax a copy of the future test results to my business phone.

The next week I stood in front of the fax machine at our shop and watched it print the lab report. My jaw dropped. Nauseated, I slumped into a chair, studied the paper, then called Jeremiah with the bad news.

Jeremiah answered the phone. Landon cried in the background.

"What's wrong?" I said.

"Shelly's changing his diaper."

I cleared my throat. "I've got the test results. The bilirubin doubled."

"Oh my gosh, that's bad. Call the transplant doctor in Boston and talk to him, then call me later and let me know what he thinks we should do. A new nurse is here, and we're getting ready to do a line change. We've got our hands full with Landon right now."

The new nurse had just joined Landon's team. The first nurse quit after a faulty blood sugar test resulted in an ambulance rushing to Jeremiah's house and scaring all of us half to death.

While they got acquainted and tended to Landon, I called the transplant doctor, who referred me to the doctor overseeing the Omegaven study. Both agreed with our conclusion—the lipids were damaging Landon's liver. Without intervention, his liver would fail soon. He needed to go to Boston for treatment and possible inclusion in the Omegaven study.

On Friday, almost three weeks after Landon came home, his surgeon sent a request to Medicaid for approval to send him to Boston. We thought that with the doctor's recommendation, taking Landon to Boston was a foregone conclusion. All we needed was a date so we could book the airline tickets.

I searched web sites for affordable flights and hotel rooms all day Saturday. Several times Jeremiah and I talked on the phone about the cost and other possible ways to get Landon to Boston. The short notice made the tickets more expensive, and we didn't have much money.

On Sunday afternoon, Kathy and I took my mother for a visit with Landon. We knew her dementia and the unfamiliar surroundings would eventually make her confused and agitated, but we wanted her to at least have some time with her great-grandson.

He didn't seem sick, yet we couldn't help but notice the yellow tint around his eyes and in his cheeks, a visible sign of liver problems.

"We've got to get him to Boston soon," I said.

Mom sat on the sofa beside Landon, and Kathy placed him in her arms. She smiled and talked in short bursts of baby talk to her great-grandson, "Tic-tic-tickle," and "Get-get-get-him," while she wiggled her finger in front of his face and touched his chin. Landon giggled and cooed.

A few minutes later, Kathy held Landon.

Kathy tried to entertain both my mother and Landon, while Jeremiah, Shelly, and I discussed the trip to Boston.

She succeeded for an hour then said, "Your mom is standing beside the car with her pocketbook in her hand. We've got to take her home."

We walked to the front porch. I looked at my mother, shook my head, then hugged my son. "Call me as soon as you hear from Medicaid and get an admission date from Boston. I'll book the flights."

During the drive home, Kathy and I listened to my mother tell us several times—at least five—about her precious great-grandson. I glanced at Mom's face in the rearview mirror. Tears filled her eyes, yet she smiled while she talked.

Monday, Jeremiah called me with bad news. His voice quivered, "Medicaid has denied our request. They won't let us take Landon to Boston. They said the FDA hadn't approved Omegaven, and it's considered an experimental treatment. They won't pay for it and won't pay to send him there for any other treatment."

I shook my head. "What are they going to do? Just let his liver go bad?"

"Yes. That's what Medicaid is going to do."

I raised my voice, "That's not right,"

"The admissions office in Boston called me with the news," Jeremiah said. "There's no appeal process, but they said they'd continue to work on Landon's case."

I took a deep breath and exhaled. "I'm going to call the admissions office back. Maybe they can tell us if there's more we can do."

During the next few days, Jeremiah and I each talked with the three ladies in Boston that we called the admissions team. They worked for the hospital and the Center for Advanced Intestinal Rehabilitation. The team had fought similar battles with other states, and they worked on the initial paperwork sent to Medicaid of North Carolina requesting treatment for Landon in Boston. We looked to them for guidance.

"I'm going to call the television stations and newspapers and go public with Medicaid's decision," I said during a call. "Imagine the headlines, MEDICAID DENIES INFANT LIFESAVING TREATMENT."

"Don't do that," the team advised. "Medicaid could harden their stance and force you to take the case to court and get a judge to make a decision. The legal process could take weeks or months. Landon may not have that much time."

It seemed going public might be an option, but only as a last resort.

The admissions team in Boston gave me two other courses of action to take before going to that extreme: First, send a letter explaining Landon's situation and the need for treatment in Boston to our State Representatives. Ask for urgent intervention in the Medicaid decision. Second, search for a legal team to represent Landon in case we needed to file a motion in court.

I thought of the third course of action. I didn't believe the person at Medicaid who denied Landon's treatment understood the situation and what we requested. If I could talk with that person, maybe I could convince them to reverse the decision.

After a considerable amount of investigating and promising not to disclose how I obtained the phone number, I called the Medicaid officer. What followed was one of the most intense, emotional phone calls of my life.

In a harsh tone, the Medicaid officer said, "How did you get this number?"

Afraid the person would hang up, I spoke fast. "Please listen to me." I swallowed hard and continued. "My grandson will die if we don't get him to Boston. The lipids are destroying his liver. Please help us."

This person held my grandson's life in their hands. My body trembled, and I couldn't breathe.

The Medicaid officer said, "The FDA has not approved Omegaven. I can't authorize experimental treatment."

I took a breath, held the cordless phone tight against my ear, leaned forward on the shop desk, and made my pitch. "It's not just the Omegaven. Every doctor involved in Landon's case, and our family, believes he needs to go to Boston for treatment. The Center for Advanced Intestinal Rehabilitation is the best in the country at treating children in Landon's condition."

I heard a long sigh.

"Medicaid of North Carolina does not have an agreement

with the State of Massachusetts to pay for the medical services you have requested. I can't authorize it."

My voice quivered, I struggled to get the words out. "We can't let my grandson's liver go bad. He'll die."

"We can send your grandson to Cincinnati for a transplant evaluation. North Carolina has an agreement with Ohio."

I tried not to sound angry, even though I was. "It's not time yet. Landon is not big enough to survive a transplant."

"Then we'll have to wait until he is."

I held the phone with both hands to keep from dropping it. "My grandson may not survive that long. Boston can save him."

Heavy breathing from the Medicaid officer made me wonder if the person was angry or maybe searching for the right words. Then, a bit of compassion in the voice, "I'm a grandparent also. I feel for you, but there's nothing more I can do."

I hung up the phone. Adrenaline jolted my body. I trembled while I pounded the arms of my office chair. The release of anger allowed me to refocus on solving the problem. I had to find a way to get Landon to Boston and the treatment he needed. His face, a tint of yellow, flashed in my mind.

Late that night, I wrote a letter explaining Landon's situation and asking for help. I addressed copies to our State Representatives, Congressional Representatives, and Senators. The next morning, I drove to the post office and handed the letters to the postmaster.

During the next few days, the responses came in the form

of calls and emails. All offered sympathy and compassion. None provided an immediate resolution. I needed to pursue the other avenue the team in Boston suggested.

I called several law firms in Raleigh and asked if they would take Landon's case and fight Medicaid. They said it would take time, and we would need to discuss the cost. That route didn't seem like an option. We didn't have time or money.

On Saturday, June 6, feeling frustrated, I made a post to the blog and disclosed the Medicaid decision. I asked for prayers. Several followers responded and prayed, while others expressed outrage.

Monday, I got a call from a young man who had been in our Scout troop fifteen years earlier. I had counseled him as he advanced to the rank of Eagle. Now a lawyer, he worked for a prestigious North Carolina law firm. He told me he had discussed Landon's case with his firm. They agreed to file motions on Landon's behalf, pro-bono. I thanked him and told him I needed to talk with Jeremiah, the team in Boston, and Landon's surgeon, and I would let him know when to proceed with filing any motions.

We continued to wait for responses from the state representatives. The team from Boston continued to negotiate with Medicaid of North Carolina. Two more days passed, and we didn't hear anything.

We were running out of options. On Wednesday, I gave the phone number for the Medicaid officer to Jeremiah and told him to call. What could it hurt? We had to try everything.

To hear Jeremiah tell it, he also made an emotional plea to Medicaid and begged the person to reverse the decision. Again, the same person refused.

On Friday, my fax machine printed the test results of the bloodwork for the week. I sat in a chair beside Kathy's sewing machine and shared the results with her.

"His bilirubin is four times the normal level. How can he survive this?" I felt defeated. What else could I do? As hard as I tried to control the situation, my grandson's fate was not in my hands.

Kathy placed her hand over mine. "Let's pray for him."

We did then wiped our tears and hugged.

"God will take care of him," Kathy said.

Saturday, I prepared for a week of Cub Scout camp at Raven Knob Scout Reservation. Our Pack had booked the time at camp, months earlier. I first camped at Raven Knob when Jeremiah was a scout, twenty years earlier. This year, with my mind on Landon and the fight to get him to Boston, I found it challenging to get ready for the trip. I moped around with my head hung while I loaded camping gear in my truck. As the leader of the Pack, and with a couple of dozen young scouts, including my grandsons Gavin and Ezekiel, eager to go camping, I had no choice but to go.

On Sunday, in my truck, I escorted a caravan of excited young scouts, parents, and leaders to camp. After we settled into our campsite, I took our Pack, most of whom had not been to Raven Knob, on a walking tour of the sprawling reservation.

During the tour, with my mind on Landon, I talked with another leader, Scott, about the battle with Medicaid. I needed to vent. Scott listened. At the time, I didn't realize how God led me to Scott and the importance of our conversation.

The next day Scott, who had returned home and to work, called Wil, a friend from his childhood Scout Troop. Wil was in the North Carolina House of Representatives and was serving on the Health and Human Services Committee, which oversaw Medicaid of North Carolina. Scott told Wil Landon's story.

Tuesday morning, unaware of Scott's conversation with Wil, I helped the other leaders get the boys off to their activities for the day. Afterward, we sat around a picnic table, under a shelter, and sipped coffee while a light rain fell. My cell phone rang.

I didn't have good phone reception at camp, yet I heard Jeremiah's voice crack, "Medicaid approved our request."

I walked out of the camp and into the forest, still thinking I missed something because of the weak phone signal. "What did you say?"

"Medicaid has agreed to send Landon to Boston."

My heart skipped a beat. I listened and stumbled into the forest, looking for higher ground and better reception. "How? What happened?" A steady rain fell. A low rumble of thunder rolled across the mountains.

"I don't know. The admissions office in Boston called me with the news." He cried. "They are talking with Medicaid, working out the details. We need to book flights to Boston, and Dad, we want you to go with us."

I breathed deep, "I'll be home in a couple of hours."

My legs trembled. I leaned against a wet tree to catch my balance, raised my hands, and looked toward the sky. "Thank you, God." Raindrops washed teardrops from my cheeks.

We're taking Landon to Boston.

Chapter 13

Boston

I delegated my responsibilities to the other Scout leaders, jumped in my truck, slapped the steering wheel, and shouted, "Yeehaw, Boston, here we come." Now, we had to find a way to get him there.

I arrived home Tuesday afternoon and called Jeremiah. "What do I need to do?"

My son answered excitedly. "The admissions office called back. We need to get Landon to Boston by next Monday, June 22. I'm searching for airline flights. Will you search for hotel rooms and figure the cost of food and cab fares?"

We talked three more times that afternoon, discussed what we found, and calculated the expense. With each conversation, our exuberance deflated more. We didn't have enough money.

"We need another thousand dollars," Jeremiah said.

I scratched my head. How could we come up with the money? "Maybe we can drive," I said.

"It's 800 miles to Boston. Your Chrysler is too small. Our Lincoln is too old. If Landon gets sick along the way, we might not find a hospital that will know how to treat him."

Out of curiosity, I researched renting a vehicle and calculated it would cost almost as much as buying airplane tickets. Driving was not the best option.

I couldn't borrow money from a bank. I had maxed out our credit a few months earlier for a business loan. Instead, maybe I could sell something. But, I couldn't think of anything I could part with worth a thousand dollars.

I stared out the window of our shop while cars zoomed by on Main Street. The gears in my mind churned. I turned to Kathy. "What do we have on the books we can reupholster and get paid for fast?"

She thumbed through the pages of the notebook we used to schedule our work. "We have a lot of work booked. But nothing we can get paid for this week."

I slumped in a chair, leaned my head back, looked at the ceiling, and whispered a prayer, "God, help us find the money we need."

I had seen God at work in Landon's life, but I hadn't discovered how to have in-depth conversations with Him. That would come much later. I did develop the practice of praying short, whispered prayers, often. I still do.

The shop phone rang. A female customer said, "I have a sofa and chair I need to have reupholstered. I have company coming this weekend. How much will it cost? Can you do it in the next couple of days?"

"The labor is one thousand dollars," I said and held my breath.

"Okay. Can you come and get it?"

One thousand dollars, exactly what we needed for the trip to Boston. "Thank you," I whispered.

I called Jeremiah and told him about the new customer.

During the next two and a half days, Kathy and I reupholstered the furniture. Friday at noon, I delivered the sofa and chair to a happy customer and collected the thousand dollars. Again, God provided what we needed.

Sunday, June 21, about 11:00 a.m., Kathy pulled the Lincoln Continental into the drop-off lane at the departure terminal of the airport in Charlotte and opened the trunk. I jumped out and removed our five suitcases.

The traffic surrounding us was chaotic.

Jeremiah pulled Landon, in his carrier, from the back seat. Shelly handed Jeremiah the bag with the pumps and the tubes connected to Landon.

Cars passed us on the left. A cab pulled in front of us.

Kathy hugged Jeremiah and Shelly and kissed Landon. She looked at me, and her eyes filled with tears. "You make sure they take care of him in Boston."

I kissed her and closed the trunk.

She jumped in the car and sped away.

The exhaust fumes and the ninety-degree heat stifled me. It couldn't be good for Landon. Barely able to breathe, I pointed at Jeremiah and Shelly. Over the engine noises and the horns beeping, I shouted, "You two get Landon inside. I'll take care of the luggage."

I struggled, but loaded our suitcases on a buggy and pushed it to the airline check-in counter.

Jeremiah and Shelly, with Landon, stood at the end of a line that led to airport security.

Less than eight years after the 9/11 attacks, we were flying to Boston and the same airport where two of the four hijacked flights originated. With security still tight, the Transportation Security Administration (TSA) banned most liquids from carry-ons.

Anxious about getting through security with suitcases packed with bags of TPN and medicines, Jeremiah approached the inspector. He presented a letter written by Landon's doctor. The letter explained the need for the TPN and the reason we must keep the fluids with us. We couldn't check the bags and take a chance on losing the TPN. Without it, Landon's blood sugar would drop. He could go into shock and die.

The TSA inspector placed the bags on a table and unzipped them. He didn't touch anything but looked at us with suspicion. I became nervous at the thought the inspector might delay us or stop us from boarding the plane. He read the letter, talked with

Jeremiah, looked at Landon, the tubes, and the pumps, then motioned for us to proceed. I exhaled.

On the airplane, I sat in a window seat—Jeremiah, Shelly, and Landon behind me. I turned around and snapped a couple of pictures of the three. Two-month-old Landon, dressed in an orange and white striped onesie, squirmed in Shelly's arms. A clear tape held the central line tube to his bare right thigh. The tube entered the pump bag tucked beside Jeremiah in his seat. Landon turned his head, looked at the bright porthole window, and closed his eyes. Soon after take-off, he fell asleep and didn't wake until we reached Boston.

We touched down to a rainy, sixty-degree afternoon. Thankfully, we brought jackets.

While Shelly rushed Landon to a bathroom for a diaper change, Jeremiah watched our luggage. I retrieved our bags, stacked them on a buggy, and knelt beside Jeremiah to catch my breath. "I'm glad I came. Traveling with Landon and all this luggage is difficult, even for three people."

The next morning our skilled cab driver negotiated the congested city traffic and drove us to the entrance of Boston Children's Hospital. The morning rush in our little hometown lasts about ten minutes - I held my breath all during the drive.

I snapped Jeremiah, Shelly, and Landon's picture in front of the hospital logo—a cameo of a nurse with a baby in her arms. I couldn't stop smiling.

A woman behind an information counter gave us directions

to the pediatric floor for small-bowel children.

"Can you believe it," I said to my son and daughter-in-law, "they have part of a floor dedicated for small-bowel children, like Landon? We came to the right place."

A nurse met us at the information desk on Landon's floor. With outstretched arms, she said, "Is this Landon?" She leaned forward and rubbed his cheek with the palm of her hand. "Come with me. I have a room prepared for you."

Landon smiled, so did I.

With Shelly's help, the nurse placed Landon in his bed, removed his pumps from the travel bag, and placed them on a pole beside his bed. "He looks good. Most children come here already near death. I see a little yellow in his face. Not much. It's good you got him here before his liver failed."

I smiled, sat in a chair, and listened to Jeremiah, Shelly, and the nurse talk about the central line, the TPN, the schedule, and the diaper rash. I marveled at the competence of the nurse. She understood what Jeremiah and Shelly talked about and knew as much, if not more, about Landon's condition than we did. Her smile told me she loved her work and the children.

Someone knocked on the door. A man in a white coat stepped in, the transplant doctor that Jeremiah and Shelly spoke with soon after Landon's birth. Without his willingness to talk with us and his recommendation, Landon would have died. Jeremiah shook his hand. I felt like wrapping my arms around him and giving him a big hug. Instead, tears filled my eyes. I smiled, grabbed his hand,

and shook.

I think our display of emotion surprised the doctor.

He stammered a few words. "I'm happy to do it." Then he examined Landon and commented about how good he looked. The doctor asked Jeremiah and Shelly about their concerns.

Jeremiah showed the doctor the red, blistered, oozing skin around the central line access site in Landon's thigh. "We think he is allergic to the adhesives in the tape and bandages, but we can't find another way to keep the central line sealed."

The doctor said, "We've got some different bandages we can try. We don't want this to get infected."

Again, someone knocked on the door. Three ladies dressed in office attire stepped in—the admissions team. It was the same threesome who had helped us in our fight with Medicaid.

The first woman turned to me. "We came to see Landon, but we also wanted to meet all of you. We haven't seen parents or grandparents fight any harder than you did to get Landon here. We don't think Medicaid would have reversed the decision without your tenacity. Somehow you made it happen."

One of the women dabbed the corner of her eye with the back of her index finger.

My throat tightened. I struggled to talk. "We didn't do it. All of us did." I pointed my finger at my son, daughter-in-law, the transplant doctor, the admissions team, then to the ceiling. "God did it."

The second woman said, "Your successful efforts have opened the door for other children from North Carolina, on Medicaid, to come to Boston Children's Hospital if they need to. We thank you."

"We have more good news," the third woman said. "The Yawkey Family Inn has granted you a room. It's a boarding house for families of patients at the hospital. They finished renovations, and you will be one of the first boarders. You can visit the house this afternoon. It's within walking distance of the hospital."

A couple of hours later, I stood on the sidewalk in front of a large Victorian house with my hand on my son's shoulder. "You and Shelly have a nice place to stay when I leave. God has provided for us again."

Boston felt right. While I walked through the city with my son, I sensed it. We did the best thing for Landon by bringing him here. The doctors in Boston would help him.

In the evening, the doctor who administered the Omegaven study came to Landon's room.

I rose from a chair, shook his hand, and thanked him for his efforts on Landon's behalf.

The doctor with salt-and-pepper hair and mustache smiled while he examined Landon. The look on his face turned serious. "Landon's bilirubin has dropped. It's below the threshold where we can give him Omegaven."

I shook my head. "That's good news. But how did it happen?"

The doctor shrugged his shoulders. He didn't have an answer, but somehow Landon's liver recovered, at least a little.

Jeremiah stood at the foot of the bed with both hands on the footboard. "What does that mean for Landon now?"

"We have already enrolled him in the study. We will test to determine how much we can reduce the lipids without harming him. And, we'll monitor him as a patient who doesn't receive Omegaven. But, if his bilirubin rises again, even though Medicaid won't pay for it, Omegaven is there for him."

I said, "What else can you do for Landon here in Boston?"

"We've scheduled a series of tests. The tests will take several days to complete but will establish a baseline for Landon and help us determine how to treat him."

The next morning, a female doctor from the Harvard School of Medicine examined Landon's organs with an ultrasound. The doctor pointed out several things about his liver to the half dozen students who watched with us.

She pointed to the red and blue colors on the screen. "This shows us partial blockages in the liver."

The doctor described it as the lipids "gunking-up" the ducts and vessels within the liver.

In the days that followed, the doctors conducted several more tests, including a test to determine how much nutrition Landon's body required and how much he absorbed through his stomach and duodenum. They also examined his heart, brain, and kidneys.

I booked a return flight to leave on Wednesday evening. I'm a history buff and couldn't leave Boston without a visit to the historic district. Wednesday morning, I took my first subway ride, went to the middle of town, and walked the Freedom Trail through light rain. The rain couldn't dampen my mood. But cobblestones get slick when wet. I landed on my back in the middle of the street in front of Paul Revere's house. We won a battle by getting Landon to Boston, but our war continued. Slightly wounded—mostly my pride—I limped back to the subway and to the hospital to say goodbye.

I held Landon in my arms and hugged him. "Your grandmother said for me to give you a kiss from her before I leave." I did.

I hugged my son and daughter-in-law. "The doctors will take care of Landon. God will take care of you." I handed Jeremiah the cash in my wallet, two hundred dollars. "Call me if you need more."

The first trip to Boston took all our savings and all the cash we could scrape up. Landon needed to return every other month until he grew big enough for a transplant.

We needed a lot more money. Eager to get home and back to work, I left the hospital and took a cab to the airport.

Chapter 14

Finances and Emergency on an Airplane

The trip to Boston didn't go the way we thought it would. We took Landon there to receive Omegaven. That didn't happen. Again, God had a different plan.

We depleted most of our funds to get Landon to Boston and weren't sure if we had enough money to bring him home.

At home, I returned to work.

Our business provided Kathy and me with a living. We even made enough to help our son and daughter-in-law keep their household running while they took care of Landon. But we didn't make enough money to fund the campaign to save Landon's life. We needed to support our family and, at the same time, find another way to raise funds for our grandson.

With school out for the summer, Ezekiel stayed at our home

with Kathy while his parents were in Boston. Roger stayed with a family friend in Taylorsville.

On my first day home, Ezekiel accompanied us to our shop and played a video game while Kathy and I worked. In the afternoon, his Aunt Jessica took him to the community swimming pool to swim with her sons, Gavin and Braiden.

That evening, after work, I stopped by my mother's apartment. She sat on the sofa, looked at a piece of paper, and cried.

"What's wrong, Mom?"

"My checking account is overdrawn." She handed me the notice.

Twenty years earlier, when my father died, my mother became an independent woman. She worked for several years and supported herself before she became eligible to draw Social Security and my father's Army pension. She took great pride in not asking her children for help. Now, at the age of seventy-five, often in a confused state of mind, she couldn't keep her checkbook balanced and occasionally ran out of money before the end of the month.

"Don't worry. I'll take care of your checking account tomorrow."

The next morning, I went to the bank and got everything straightened out.

Saturday morning, June 27, Kathy and I went back to work. Something we usually didn't do on the weekend. The phone rang. I rushed to the desk and answered.

Jeremiah, with panic in his voice, said, "Something's wrong with Landon. His right leg is swelling. There might be a leak in his central line. They took him to an exam room to run a dye through the central line and do an ultrasound. I'll call back as soon as we know more."

Careful not to alarm Ezekiel, who had accompanied us to work again, Kathy and I held hands and prayed a silent prayer for Landon.

Two hours later, Jeremiah called back. "He has a blood clot around his central line." My son gasped. "The doctor said if they can't get the clot dissolved soon enough, Landon could lose his leg." He sniffled, and his voice quivered. "If the blood clot breaks loose and travels to his heart, he'll die. He's getting a blood thinner through an IV line."

Had Landon been close enough, Kathy and I would have jumped in the car and raced to the hospital, but he was 800 miles away. We couldn't do that. So, we held each other, cried, and prayed again.

I returned to work, but the thoughts of Landon losing a leg or worse, dying, made it difficult to focus. The head of the hammer landed squarely on my thumbnail. I shouted in pain, grabbed my thumb, and sat in a chair.

Kathy, cheery and pleasant, yet with tears in her eyes, waited on a customer who was shopping for fabric.

During the next few hours, we listened for the phone to ring and jumped when it did.

"The clot is dissolving, and the swelling is going down," Jeremiah said, the relief evident in his voice.

The blood clot happened in a hospital where the doctors knew how to handle the situation; anywhere else, and he might have died. This time I didn't whisper. I looked at the ceiling and said, "Thank you, God."

On Monday, the short-bowel doctor proposed a different course of action. He wanted to stop the TPN for several hours each day. He called this "cyclic TPN." He reasoned that Landon's liver had shown a remarkable ability to heal itself. Stopping the TPN for short periods might give his liver time to clean itself out and prevent liver damage.

The doctor's recommendation created a new procedure for Jeremiah and Shelly to learn—how to fill the line with an anti-clotting solution and then cap it. The doctor recommended another change, pumping more formula into Landon's stomach.

One of the tests from the previous week indicated Landon could metabolize a little nutrition through what remained of his digestive system. To take advantage of the discovery, the doctor ordered more feeding through the G-tube. The more nutrition Landon could take in, the faster he would gain weight, and the sooner he could get a transplant. But continuous pump feeding would increase the need for diaper changes and exacerbate the problem with the diaper rash. Even so, willing to do anything to give their son an advantage, Jeremiah and Shelly agreed.

In Boston, diaper changes, formula changes, cycling the TPN, and walking to the Yawkey Family Inn, filled their days. Jeremiah and Shelly took turns at the Inn, much like they did at the Ronald McDonald House in Winston-Salem. Shelly stayed at the hospital most nights and Jeremiah on most days.

Thursday afternoon, July 2—Kathy's birthday, with the blood clot completely dissolved and no more tests to do, Jeremiah and Shelly convinced the doctor they could cycle the TPN and care for Landon at home. After ten days in Boston, the doctor agreed to discharge him.

Jeremiah called our shop phone with the good news. "Happy birthday, Mom. If we can get a flight out, we are coming home tomorrow."

Kathy let out a "Woohoo" and pumped her fist in the air. "We finished a big job this week, and the money is in the bank. Go ahead and book a flight. We'll meet you at the airport in Charlotte. And thanks, this is the best birthday present ever." After the call, Kathy, usually a little more reserved, danced around our shop with her hands over her head, singing, "Landon's coming home. Landon's coming home."

The doctors discharged Landon the next day. To continue the scheduled cycle, Jeremiah stopped the TPN before they left Boston. He planned to restart it after they arrived in Charlotte. We didn't know how long Landon could remain off the TPN until his blood sugar would drop, but if everything went as planned, they should have plenty of time to get to Charlotte and get it restarted before that happened.

Jeremiah and Shelly got to the airport early, but unfortunately, the plane left a few minutes late.

Before Kathy and I went to the airport to meet the flight, we rendezvoused with a courier from the pharmacy at Jeremiah and Shelly's home. He had a week's supply of Landon's TPN. We put most in the refrigerator but took one bag with us to the airport. Jeremiah planned to use the bag to reconnect Landon's TPN when they arrived.

The plane landed in Charlotte to a busy airport and ninety-five-degree heat. They remained in the airplane, waiting to taxi to a gate. This airline must not have had enough gate space or high priority to get one. Thirty minutes passed on the hot tarmac.

Inside the stuffy plane, drenched with sweat, Jeremiah called me. "Dad, we're stuck on this hot airplane. The pilot announced that we are waiting for a gate."

Kathy and I stood at the top of the escalator that led to baggage claim, where we had agreed to meet Jeremiah, Shelly, and Landon.

Another thirty minutes passed. I called Jeremiah's phone, but it went straight to voicemail.

I nudged Kathy's shoulder with my elbow. "This is bad. They've got to hook Landon's TPN back up."

She placed a cupped hand over her mouth and nodded.

Fifteen minutes later, I called Jeremiah. Again, voicemail. "I don't understand. He should answer or call back."

Almost an hour and a half after the plane landed, I spotted an emergency cart approaching us from Concourse B. Shelly sat in the front seat and held Landon in her arms.

"Here they come." I waved my hand in the air and shouted, "We're over here."

Jeremiah sat in the rear seat and faced away. He held their carry-on luggage and the infant carrier. The driver pulled the cart in front of us and stopped. Shelly stepped off.

Landon's left arm dangled at his side, and his eyes stared at the ceiling. He didn't react to us or anything around him. I wondered if we were already too late.

"His sugar must be low," Jeremiah said. "We've got to get his TPN started."

"Oh my gosh, look how pale he is," Kathy said. "Follow me."

At the bottom of the escalator, everyone but me bolted toward the exit.

I shouted, "Jeremiah, how many bags do you have?"

"Four." He raised his hand, showed four fingers, and continued out the door.

I went to baggage claim and retrieved their luggage.

At the car, Kathy removed the TPN from a cooler in the trunk. In the backseat, Jeremiah did his best to create a sterile environment with changing pads. Sweat dripped in his eyes while he connected the TPN line and started the pumps.

I loaded the luggage in the trunk, climbed in the driver's seat, cranked the car, and turned the air conditioner on. While the car cooled, we sat in silence, all eyes on Landon, watching for signs of improvement, willing him to come around. I still thought we might need to take him to a hospital.

In the back seat, Shelly held Landon in her arms. Little by little, the color returned to his cheeks. He turned his head, looked at his mother, and smiled.

She hugged him. With his face close to hers, she said, "He's okay."

I shifted the car into drive and headed for Jeremiah and Shelly's home, an hour away. During the ride, they told us what happened on the plane after their cell phone battery died.

Shelly said that about an hour after the plane arrived, Landon became lethargic. She noticed a glazed-over look about his eyes. When she gently shook him, and he didn't respond the way he usually would, she grabbed Jeremiah's arm and said, "Something's wrong."

Jeremiah waved his hand. A female flight attendant noticed, and after she approached, he explained the situation. The attendant told him to stay calm. Backing away, she added that they would get a gate soon.

Jeremiah raised his voice. "No, you don't understand. We need to get our son off this plane now."

Shelly held Landon and cried.

Another attendant joined the discussion, then went to the cockpit. When she returned with the pilot, Jeremiah retrieved the doctor's letter and showed it to the pilot.

"My son could die on this airplane. If he does, I'll hold this airline responsible."

The pilot read the letter, looked at Landon, and at the central line taped to his thigh. He returned to the cockpit, and within minutes the pilot taxied the plane to the gate of another airline. Jeremiah, Shelly, and Landon deplaned first. An emergency cart was waiting, and the driver brought them to where we waited at the top of the escalator.

When Jeremiah and Shelly finished telling us the story, I looked at Kathy sitting in the front passenger seat. A tear rolled down her cheek. For the next hour, we rode in silence. Jeremiah, Shelly, and Landon dozed in the back seat.

The trip revealed Landon's fragility and how fast the situation can turn bad.

Even with the medical scares and the financial problems, we considered the trip to Boston a success. Omegaven was available for Landon if he needed it, and the doctors started him on a path focused on saving his liver and helping him grow big enough for a transplant as soon as possible.

The doctor in Boston scheduled another appointment for August 13, six weeks away. Not much time to come up with the money for another trip. And this was a huge factor; he also would need to return every six to eight weeks.

We had to find a way to finance the trips and get him there and back, safely.

Chapter 15

COTA

Taking charity is not in my nature. However, I would do anything to get a life-saving transplant for Landon, even asking other people for money. But I couldn't ask. Not yet.

If we accepted donations, the IRS required Jeremiah to report it as family income. The increase in revenue could make his son ineligible for Medicaid. Without Medicaid or private insurance—which the family couldn't afford—Landon could not get a transplant. He would die.

We had to find a way to raise money without jeopardizing my grandson's security.

We discovered two options. We could establish a trust to accept and administer the funds, or we could partner with a non-profit organization that helped families in situations like ours.

I called an attorney. She explained the complicated process of establishing a trust fund and how we would need to recruit a board of trustees. She emphasized that if we did one thing wrong, it could lead to legal, tax, and insurance issues. It didn't sound like something we wanted to do.

Early in this journey, I discovered the websites and blogs of several intestinal transplant children. The families of those children had partnered with the Children's Organ Transplant Association (COTA) to help with fundraising efforts. I called COTA, explained Landon's situation, and our dire need to raise money. The lady on the phone said they could help. She mailed an information packet, and two days later, in my shop, I studied every word. Eager to share the information with my son, I called.

"There's more here than we can discuss on the phone. If we decide to partner with COTA, you and Shelly will sign a contract. I need to show you this packet."

"Shelly's grandparents want us to go to church with them tomorrow morning," Jeremiah said. "Why don't you and Mom drive down and go with us? Bring the packet. After church, we'll grill hamburgers and look at the information."

The next morning Kathy and I sat in a pew with Jeremiah's family and Shelly's grandparents during Sunday morning services at the Stony Point Baptist Church. Kathy and I hadn't attended a church service in a long time.

The worship and the sermon stirred something in me. I resolved to find a church near our home and attend more often.

After the service, we thanked the pastor again for all his prayers.

That afternoon, at our son's home, hamburgers sizzled on the grill while Ezekiel enjoyed a tree swing, and Kathy pushed Landon in a baby stroller around the shady yard until he needed a diaper change. I followed her into the house to get a cold soft drink from the refrigerator. Landon wailed when Kathy wiped his bottom.

Like before, she whispered, "I'm sorry, I'm sorry." She held a large tube of white cream. "The doctors in Boston gave them this cream for the diaper rash. It helps when they use a lot of it." She smeared a thick layer of the white ointment on Landon's bottom then fastened the fresh diaper. With him snug in her arms and a pacifier in his mouth, Kathy rocked and hummed. Soon Landon slept.

Jeremiah, Shelly, and I sat around a picnic table, looked at the information in the packet, and talked about COTA.

Several things about this organization appealed to us. First, it only assisted families of children in need of a transplant. Having helped other families like ours, COTA would understand our needs. Second, they did not use any of the funds raised for the children to cover administrative costs. Other organizations did. All the money donated in honor of Landon would go toward transplant-related expenses, nothing else. Employees of COTA and volunteers raised funds needed for the administrative cost through other means—charity events, donations, etc.

COTA would establish and administer a tax-exempt trust account for Landon and provide a website for fundraising. I liked the promise of logistical support, advice for fundraising events, and oversight of our activities. With help from COTA, we could raise money and avoid trouble with the IRS and Medicaid.

After we ate hamburgers and hot dogs, we talked for a couple more hours. My son and daughter-in-law decided to partner with COTA.

July 15, 2011, *The Alleghany News*, our local newspaper, published an article about Landon and our efforts to get him a transplant. In the article, we announced an organizational meeting for those interested in volunteering for the fundraising campaign.

Sunday, July 19, at 2:00 p.m., we met with a COTA representative and a group of eager volunteers in the fellowship hall of the First Baptist Church in Sparta. Jeremiah and Shelly made the one-hour drive from their home in Taylorsville and brought Landon.

Many of the volunteers met our precious grandson for the first time at the meeting. I heard a lot of "oohs" and "aahs." Landon smiled and soaked up the love.

For several days before the meeting, I worked to produce a thirty-minute video about Landon. Kathy and Shelly brought baked goods for refreshments. Our family and the two dozen in attendance settled into chairs behind white folding tables. I dimmed the lights and pressed play on the DVD player. We watched a television atop a rolling cart and nibbled on sweets. Half-way through the video, someone behind me sniffled. A woman beside me reached for a napkin on the table and dabbed her eyes. The video ended with me telling how Landon couldn't survive without a transplant and why we needed to raise money for transplant-related expenses. I flipped on the lights and stood before the crowd. Several volunteers wiped tears from their cheeks.

I gave them a moment to compose themselves before I said, "We have determined that our family needs to raise $75,000 to help Landon get a transplant."

One lady near the front placed her hand over her mouth. There were wide eyes and raised eyebrows.

I took a deep breath. $75,000 might not seem like a lot of money to some, but to our community, it was.

"We have help," I said, trying to reassure the volunteers. "A lady from the Children's Organ Transplant Association is here to help us get organized and get started." I introduced the COTA representative, who had flown in from Indiana.

The lady stepped to the podium. She told us about a little boy whose liver failed. The family of the sick child raised money for a transplant, but he died before he received one. After the child's death, the family donated the money to establish COTA and help other families in similar situations.

After telling us how COTA got started, the lady helped us organize our fundraising team. We decided who would do what.

Then, Jeremiah, his eyebrows furrowed, said, "How can we raise that much money?"

The representative smiled, "I suggest you begin with a coin box campaign."

She held a six-inch cardboard cube in her hands. "This is a

coin box. Volunteers place these boxes in stores. Customers put their change in it."

"Do you expect us to raise $75,000 one quarter at a time?" asked a volunteer.

"You've got to start somewhere," the COTA representative said.

Trying not to show my skepticism, I smiled.

The lady pointed to a stack of flat cardboard on a table. "There are about fifty boxes in this stack. You need to assemble them, take them to local stores, and place them on the checkout counters, near the cash registers."

Monday morning, at our shop, I assembled the preprinted boxes. "Help Make a Miracle for a family in this community, Children's Organ Transplant Association, and Giving Hope ... Making Miracles" was printed in blue on the front of the white boxes. I felt like we needed more. So, I glued a picture of Landon's little face to each box, with the words, "Be a Ray of Hope for Landon Joines. Landon needs a life-saving small-bowel transplant" printed above the picture.

I hoped the picture would evoke an emotional response. Who wouldn't want to help a cute, sick baby? For two days, several hours each day, I assembled boxes and numbered each one.

Wednesday evening, three volunteers met with me at our shop. We loaded boxes in our vehicles. I gave each volunteer a sheet of paper and a pen so they could record the box number, the store name, and the location where they left a box. We decided on the routes each of us would take and headed out. At each stop, we told the store manager Landon's story and asked if we could leave a box. Most agreed. The stores that didn't were owned by corporations and didn't allow such things in their businesses.

At one small neighborhood convenience store, the owner—a man with olive-toned skin, listened while I told Landon's story. He didn't smile. When I finished, I expected to hear him say "no." Instead, he reached in his pocket, pulled out a $100 bill, and handed it to me. With a Middle Eastern accent, he said, "This is for your grandson. Place the box by the cash register." I didn't meet the man again. But, in the weeks that followed, the box at his store was among the top in donations.

We placed all the boxes we had. I ordered more.

A couple of days after we started the coin box campaign, the staff from COTA helped me prepare a media release about Landon and our fundraising efforts. They sent me a printout with the contact information of the newspapers, radio stations, and television stations in our area. I sent the media release to as many as I could.

Monday morning, July 31, our shop phone rang.

A woman said, "I'm a reporter for WXII Channel 12 News in Winston-Salem. We want to do a story about Landon for the evening news."

I caught the phone before I dropped it. "Please do." My legs wobbled, I slumped to the chair at the desk.

"We'll be there by noon," the reporter said.

The publicity could be the big break we needed for the fundraising campaign. I called Jeremiah and Shelly, then rushed home to help Kathy tidy up around the house. Our son and daughter-in-law arrived, with Landon, thirty minutes before the reporter and cameraman did.

Jeremiah and Shelly, with Landon on his mother's lap, sat close together on our sofa. The cameraman recorded while the reporter asked questions. A tear appeared in the corner of the reporter's eye. Still, she smiled when the cameraman pointed the camera at her.

Afterward, the cameraman followed me to our shop and took a video of me while I assembled coin boxes. He left in a hurry saying he needed to get back to the studio to edit the video. He also said he wanted to stop at a couple of the stores where we had placed boxes.

At 6:20 p.m., Landon's smiling face appeared on our television screen during the newscast.

"Oohah, look how cute he is," Kathy swooned.

We leaned forward.

The video zoomed out to show Landon sitting on Shelly's lap and Jeremiah beside the two. Jeremiah and Shelly told Landon's story.

The reporter said, "Local volunteers are raising money for Landon's transplant." She told the audience about the coin box campaign, then showed the video of me assembling boxes at our shop and of a box on a counter in a local store. The newscast ended with the reporter saying, "Please, help little Landon get a transplant."

Wednesday evening, two days after Landon's television debut, my phone rang.

"You need to come and get this box," the store owner said.

"Someone will be there tomorrow morning."

The next morning, I got calls from two more store owners. Both wanted us to pick up the boxes at their stores.

A few minutes before noon, a car zoomed into the parking lot of our shop and backed to the door. One of our volunteers jumped out of the car and ran into the shop. "You've got to see these boxes," she said.

Kathy and I followed her to the back of her car, where she opened the trunk revealing ten bulging boxes. The store owners didn't want us to remove the boxes. They wanted us to replace them because they were full.

Kathy leaned over the trunk and grabbed one. "It's heavy."

The outpouring of love for Landon blew us away.

Giddy, the three of us carried the boxes into the shop and laughed. After we placed the last box on the table, Kathy picked out the heaviest one and opened it. Cash fell on the table, and I threw my hands in the air, astonished. Kathy covered her mouth with her right hand. The three of us separated the money and counted.

The first box contained $107.37.

We high fived and hugged.

I looked at the other nine boxes. "We can do this," I said.

That evening, eager to check my route, I drove to the locations where I had placed boxes days ago.

While gone, the two other volunteers returned to our shop with the boxes they retrieved. Kathy and the volunteers counted and recorded. Not every box contained more than $100, but a few did.

All the coins and cash created another problem, how to get the money into Landon's COTA account. To solve the problem, COTA opened an account for Landon at a local bank where we could deposit the cash.

Friday evening, I placed a heavy bag on the counter at the bank and handed the teller a note with the account number written on it. "I need to deposit this money into this account," I said and pointed at the number on the note.

The teller frowned. "You need to roll the coins," she said while she typed the account number on her keyboard and looked at the computer screen. "Wait, this is for the little boy that needs a transplant. Isn't it?"

"Yes." I smiled. "My grandson."

Another teller walked over. "We can do it this time." She smiled and pulled the bag from the counter.

A lady in line behind me said, "I saw your grandson's story on the news."

I turned and smiled at her.

When the tellers finished counting, one announced, "$1,068.22."

She clapped and cheered, as did the other teller, and the customers behind me. I choked back a tear and left the bank with a bag of paper coin tubes.

Within a few weeks, our team circulated almost two hundred boxes across northwest North Carolina. We continued the coin box campaign until the donations dwindled. Satisfied with the results, having collected several thousand dollars, we removed the boxes.

The success of the coin box campaign jump-started our fundraising efforts and relieved some of the financial burdens of taking care of Landon. We no longer worried about where the money would come from for the next trip or the next hospital stay.

Encouraged and enthusiastic, several volunteers planned future COTA fundraising events.

I turned my attention toward solving another problem.

Chapter 16

Children's Flight of Hope

The money donated during the first week of the coin box campaign took a lot of pressure off our family. We raised enough that, had we chosen to, we could have bought the airplane tickets for the second trip to Boston. But after the medical scare on the plane during the first trip, the thoughts of flying Landon on a commercial flight again terrified us. I explored other options.

Kathy and I sat at our dining room table. The evening news played on the television in the living room. I reached over my taco salad and tapped the keys on my laptop computer.

"I wish you wouldn't mess with that thing while we're eating supper," Kathy huffed.

"I know, but I'm looking for a van or a motorhome. Maybe we can take Landon to Boston in one." I stared at the screen and munched on a mouthful of lettuce.

"We can't afford to buy another vehicle."

I knew we couldn't, but my mind churned. I wrestled with the problem of how to get Landon to Boston and back without putting him on another commercial flight.

Kathy went to the kitchen to refill her glass with sweet tea.

The reporter on the television said, "Our next story is about an organization that flies sick children to hospitals for free."

I dropped my fork, jumped from the table, and ran to the living room. Kathy came from the kitchen to see what caused the commotion. The reporter told the story of a sick child and then showed a video of pilots flying the child in a private plane to a distant hospital.

"This is it. This is what we need for Landon," I said. "Quick, get something to write on."

Kathy grabbed a notepad and pencil from the telephone table in the dining room, ran back to the living room, scribbled the contact information, and handed it to me.

I stared at the number. What just happened? The answer to my problem seemed to have dropped out of the sky.

At work the next morning, I dialed the number. A lady answered, and I spoke fast, telling her Landon's story and of our need for a flight to Boston in a few weeks.

"I'm sorry," she said. "There's no way we can help you that soon. We are booked weeks in advance, and the approval process could take more than a few weeks."

My excitement fizzled. I looked at the floor. Was this a dead end?

"Wait." She paused. "Did you say you are from North Carolina?"

"Yes," I said and raised my head.

"There's an organization in North Carolina called the Children's Flight of Hope. They might be able to help you." She gave me a phone number and wished me luck.

I hung up and dialed as fast as I could.

Another lady answered.

I started talking before I realized I had reached an answering machine. I waited for the message to end. After the beep, I said. "My grandson lives in Taylorsville and needs to go to the hospital in Boston. Please help us." I left our shop number, hoping someone would call back soon.

The rest of the day, I worked on furniture and waited for the call. I stared at the phone, willing it to ring. When it did, I jumped to answer. A customer asked for Kathy. I gave the phone to my wife and trudged back to work.

Kathy finished her work at about 4:00 p.m. and went home.

At 5:00 p.m., my hopes dashed, I decided to go home also. At the door, the phone rang. I ran to the desk and answered.

The same voice I had heard on the answering machine earlier said, "I'm with the Children's Flight of Hope. I got a message that you have a child who needs to go to Boston."

My heart thumped. I took a deep breath and blurted out Landon's story. I told the lady about our experience on the commercial flight and his next appointment in Boston.

In an encouraging tone, the lady said, "This is short notice. But I'll fax you some forms. Answer the questions on the forms and fax them back to me as soon as you can. I'll present it to our team. Maybe we can help."

A few minutes later, the fax machine beeped and printed four pages.

Since most of the questions on the forms asked about Landon's condition, the need for a flight, the family finances, and the contact information for Landon's doctors—questions I couldn't answer—I called Jeremiah. An hour later, I faxed the completed forms to The Children's Flight of Hope and raced home to share my excitement with Kathy.

The next day, a little before noon, the shop phone rang. Expecting a customer, I was startled to hear the voice of the lady from the Children's Flight of Hope. I pointed at the phone and motioned for Kathy to join me. She rushed over and placed her ear next to mine.

The excitement in the lady's voice revealed the good news. "I verified your information and talked with the doctor's office in Boston. Our team says we can do it."

Kathy stepped back and pumped her right fist in the air.

"Yes," I said, hanging up the phone. "They're going to fly Landon to Boston." I grabbed Kathy and hugged her.

She pulled back, snatched the phone from my hand, and smiled. "Let me call Jeremiah and give him the good news."

The Children's Flight of Hope agreed to fly Landon to Boston every six weeks. They also agreed to provide a rental car to get him from the airport to the hospital, and the pilots would drive them there.

August 13, about 11:00 a.m., Kathy and I met Jeremiah, Shelly, and their three boys in the parking lot of the Statesville Regional Airport. Jeremiah and the older boys unloaded the luggage from the car. Kathy helped Shelly with Landon.

"I'll go in and check on the flight," I said.

I rushed into the small lobby, not much bigger than a large living room. A driver from one of the top NASCAR teams sat alone in the waiting area. I think my sudden entrance startled him. He jumped but remained seated. We made eye contact, and I nodded. Any other time, I would have stopped and acted like a fan. Now, I was a man on a mission, and it didn't involve him. He slumped in his seat and smiled when I walked past him. I continued another thirty feet across the shiny tile floor to the information counter. "Is the Flight of Hope here yet?"

"No," the attendant standing behind the counter said. "We got a message from the airport in Raleigh. The plane left there a few minutes ago. They'll be here soon."

Shelly, with Landon in her arms, entered the terminal. The attendant smiled and pointed to a section of chairs behind the NASCAR driver. "Your family can wait there. I'll let you know when the flight arrives."

Shelly headed towards the designated waiting area with the pump bag hanging from her shoulder and tubes dangling from the bag and Landon's thigh. Kathy and Roger entered and joined Shelly. Roger pulled a rolling carry-on suitcase.

I stood at a large glass window and stared at the runway. Ezekiel ran across the waiting room and joined me. Jeremiah followed.

"Where are they?" he said in a quick, nervous tone.

"They should be here soon," I tried to sound calm and reassuring. I wasn't. Butterflies fluttered in my stomach. I focused on the activity on the apron, the area outside the terminal where planes refuel and passengers board.

Two men dressed in pilot's uniforms loaded suitcases into a private jet.

A few minutes later, the NASCAR driver boarded the jet, and we watched it take off.

About 11:30 a.m., the man behind the counter announced, "The Flight of Hope is arriving."

Ezekiel jumped and squealed the way eight-year-old boys do, "I see it, I see it." He pointed toward the end of the runway.

Soon, the small black dot grew big enough to see the shape of the approaching aircraft. The airplane touched down, zoomed along the runway past the terminal, and then slowed to a steady roll.

Compared to a commercial aircraft, this plane was small. The size of the plane did nothing to ease my fears. Still, I knew it was better than putting Landon back on a commercial flight.

The plane taxied to the apron and stopped.

Kathy took Landon from Shelly's arms and held him close. She spoke fast and jittery. "Goodbye, little man. I'll see you soon." Tears filled her eyes.

My throat tightened when Kathy handed Landon back to Shelly and hugged Jeremiah. I swallowed hard.

Unlike a large commercial airport, there were no gate agents. Jeremiah opened the door to the apron, walked through, and held it open for us.

We approached the aircraft and introduced ourselves to the two pilots. I remember thinking their grey hair gave the impression of confidence and experience. My anxiety eased a little.

We shook hands. "Please take care of my family," I said.

Before they boarded the airplane, I snapped a picture of Jeremiah, Shelly, Landon, and the two pilots.

Kathy, Roger, Ezekiel, and I returned to the terminal and watched the plane as it roared down the runway and lifted off. We waved, Ezekiel both hands as fast as he could. The plane rose above the trees to our right and turned to the north behind us. We watched and waved until it disappeared above the terminal.

Kathy wiped tears. I wrapped one arm around her shoulder and the other around Ezekiel's. "Let's go to the mountains. We have fish to catch."

An hour later, at about 1:00 p.m., we arrived home. Roger and Ezekiel grabbed fishing poles and headed for the river. It's incredible how a mountain stream stocked with trout can excite young boys. And old boys too, yet I couldn't get Jeremiah, Shelly, and Landon off my mind.

Jeremiah later told me how, having never flown in a small aircraft, it took he and Shelly a few minutes to get used to the sudden jolts and shakiness. The pilots gave them noise-canceling headphones to block the roar.

Landon rode well. When the time came for his diaper change, Shelly did it on the seat. The smell made one of the two pilots gag and dry heave. The other laughed.

At 2:56 p.m., three hours after leaving Statesville, the pilots landed at the airport in Norwood, Massachusetts, a little south of Boston. They helped Jeremiah, Shelly, and Landon to a rental car and then drove them to Boston Children's Hospital.

There, the doctors and nurses with the Center for Advanced Intestinal Rehabilitation (CAIR) examined Landon and did several tests. This clinic visit was required to keep Landon in the Omegaven study and make sure it was available for him, should his liver begin to fail. The doctors also monitored his growth, nutritional needs, and decided where to make changes in his care or his TPN formula.

The visit lasted about three hours. During this time, the pilots waited in the rental car in the hospital parking garage. Jeremiah and Shelly emerged from the hospital with Landon and returned to the car. The pilots, concerned about a line of thunderstorms brewing over the East Coast, wanted to get back to the airport and out of the Boston area before the storms arrived.

They beat the storms out of Boston, but the rains caught them in Baltimore when they stopped to refuel. The bumpy ride on the approach made Shelly airsick. Jeremiah told her to close her eyes when he realized the plane was approaching the runway sideways. The pilots executed a perfect crosswind landing in driving rain, which stopped soon after they landed.

While the pilots refueled, Jeremiah and Shelly walked around outside the plane, got some fresh air, and gave their stomachs time to stop flip-flopping. After refueling, they resumed the flight and touched down in Statesville about 1:30 a.m. Landon slept during most of the trip.

The next morning, Jeremiah called us from their home and told us how well the trip went, other than the storm in Baltimore.

Little did we know another type of storm was brewing.

Chapter 17

Lost - Alzheimer's and Central Lines

The last couple of weeks in August went well. Then came September. And the infection.

Friday afternoon, September 4, the phone rang at our shop. Jeremiah. "We think the skin around Landon's central line is infected. He has a lump in his thigh above the line. His leg is not swelling, so we don't think it's another blood clot, but we are on our way to Baptist Hospital."

I laid the staple puller in my hand on the desk. "Is he running a fever?"

Kathy saw the concern on my face, rose from the chair at her sewing machine, and rushed to my side.

"Yes, a little, his leg is warm to the touch, and he's cranky," Jeremiah said.

If Landon was "cranky"—as Jeremiah stated—he must be sick.

A few minutes later, Kathy left the shop and made the one-hour drive to Jeremiah's house. When school dismissed, she picked up Roger and Ezekiel and brought them to the mountains. I stayed on the mountain to meet with volunteers planning the next COTA fundraiser.

After work and after the meeting, I stopped by my mother's apartment. She sat on her sofa crocheting, something she had done most evenings for as long as I could remember.

Mom believed everything good that happened to her came from God, and everything bad came from the devil. This day, in a clear state of mind, she said, "God is good to me," and showed me a twenty-dollar bill she received in the mail from a friend in Florida.

"I've been praying for extra money, so I could go and see my sister, and here it is." She waved the money in my face.

I didn't argue the fact that Mom's birthday was a few weeks away and her friend sent the money as a birthday present.

"I can't take you to Aunt Jo's house tomorrow. I need to work."

Mom smiled. "That's okay. I'll drive myself."

The mother I remembered, confident and independent, emerged.

I wasn't that concerned that she wanted to drive herself to her sister's house in Laurel Springs. It was only sixteen miles away with one turn off the main road. Over the years, my mother made the trip many times by herself. She usually left early and seldom stayed for more than a few hours. Mom didn't have a cell phone. Still, I wrote my sister's phone number and my number on a piece of paper and gave it to her.

"Be careful. Call one of us from Aunt Jo's phone when you get there."

Mom put the paper and the money in her purse then laid it next to her Bible on the coffee table. "God takes care of me. He is taking care of Landon also. I've been praying for that sweet baby."

At the hospital, the doctors admitted Landon and started an antibiotic drip. A few minutes later, allergic to the antibiotic, Landon's body turned red, and hives covered his torso.

A nurse rushed in, stopped the drip, and administered an antihistamine. Afraid his throat might swell shut, the nurse stayed with Landon and monitored his breathing for several minutes. The antihistamine worked. The redness and hives went away. He breathed easy, and so did we.

The doctors waited until the next morning to administer a different antibiotic. Hopefully, one that didn't cause Landon to have an allergic reaction.

At 7:00 a.m., on my way to work, I drove by my mother's apartment. Her car was not in her parking space. As I expected, she left early to visit her sister. I worked until 5:00 p.m. and again drove past Mom's apartment before going home. She still wasn't there.

At home, concerned, I asked Kathy, "Did Mom call here today?"

"No."

I called Aunt Jo. "Has Mom left yet?"

"She didn't come here today."

"Oh, no." I slapped my forehead and hung up.

I rushed to the kitchen, where Kathy was busy cooking supper. "Mom is missing. I need to call the sheriff."

In the mountains of North Carolina, it's not unusual to hear about someone who drove off the side of a mountain, and no one found them for hours or even days. A vision of Mom's car in a ravine flashed in my mind. Nauseated, I sat in a dining chair and took deep breaths.

Kathy searched the phone book for the number to the sheriff's office. Our phone rang. I grabbed the receiver and answered—my sister.

"Mom is in Boone. A police officer called me. We are leaving now to go get her."

I plopped back into the chair, placed both elbows on the table, and cradled my head in my hands. Maybe God did take care of my mother.

As best as we could determine, Mom missed the turn to her sister's house. Unaware, she continued driving and looking for the turn. Hours later and almost eighty miles from Sparta, she saw a sign that said Tennessee; at least that's what she told the police officer. She turned around and drove back to Boone. Evening approached. Still forty miles from home, and not knowing how to get there, she stopped in the parking lot of a restaurant.

An employee found her crying, agitated, and disoriented and called for paramedics and the police. The paramedics checked her out. She hadn't eaten since breakfast, and her blood sugar was low. The restaurant employee gave her cookies and orange juice. In Mom's purse, the officer found the paper with our phone numbers on it. He called my sister.

She and my brother-in-law drove to Boone and brought Mom home.

The next morning on my way out of town to visit Landon at the hospital, I drove past mom's apartment. Surprised that she hadn't gone to church, I stopped to check on her. She smiled when I opened the door but seemed to have forgotten the ordeal from the previous day, or she didn't want to talk about it. The confident woman I spoke with two days earlier gone. Her hands shook. When I turned to leave, she followed me to the door, stuck her head out, looked around, and then shut the door and locked it. Fear now accompanied her confusion. That was the last time my mom drove out of our little town, and she seldom left her apartment.

A little before noon, in my pickup truck, I followed Kathy, Roger, and Ezekiel, who were in our car, to the hospital in Winston-Salem. Kathy planned to take the boys to their home, after we visited with Landon, and stay with them there for a few days.

Landon smiled when we entered the room. Kathy leaned over his crib and touched his arm. He giggled. He played with the toys in his bed and squealed when his two brothers played with him.

Earlier, the doctors replaced the adhesive bandage on his thigh with layers of gauze. The thick layers covered most of his thigh. Jeremiah said the nurses coated the skin around the central line with an antibiotic ointment. We hoped the cream and the antibiotics would knock out the infection.

That afternoon, Jeremiah and Shelly, wanting to spend time with their older boys, took them to a movie while Kathy and I, happy to see Landon in such a good mood, stayed at the hospital and played with our four-month-old grandson. Dressed in a blue onesie, he pointed at the small stuffed animals that circled on the crib mobile above his bed and giggled while music played. Later Kathy held him in her arms, and he sucked on a blue pacifier while they looked out the hospital window at the city below. Then I held him on my lap, and we watched television. When Jeremiah, Shelly, and the boys returned, Kathy left with Roger and Ezekiel, and I returned to the mountains.

Monday, the infection got worse. Landon's temperature rose.

Tuesday morning, Jeremiah called and told me the surgeon would remove Landon's central line in a few hours. Early on, the doctors stressed how precious each of the six central line access sites was. Now we were down to five, and we had so far to go.

On the afternoon of September 8, Kathy and I, having returned to Landon's hospital room, held each other, watched, and trembled.

Our grandson lay sideways on his bed. Jeremiah held his son's arms while Shelly stood close behind her husband. The surgeon, on the opposite side of the bed, wore a yellow sterile gown, a surgical mask, and blue latex gloves. He cleaned Landon's thigh with alcohol, then used a small syringe and administered local anesthesia around the access site. Three surgical nurses, dressed the same as the surgeon, stood with him. One held Landon's legs. A yellow mylar smiley face balloon, tied to the head of the bed, hovered above the scene.

The surgeon waited a few minutes for the medicine to numb the site, then inserted the tip of a small pair of scissors beside the tube where it entered Landon's thigh and clipped the skin. To me, Landon's ear-piercing scream meant pain. Kathy grabbed my forearm with both her hands and squeezed. Her nails dug into my flesh, and my muscles tensed.

The surgeon raised both his hands; one still held the scissors. "I promise you he is numb."

Landon whimpered.

Then, with a smooth, steady motion, the surgeon pulled the fourteen-inch line from the vein in Landon's thigh. Jeremiah, still holding his son's arms, kissed his forehead.

Shelly leaned forward and laid her head on Jeremiah's back. We cried for Landon's suffering and mourned the loss of his first central line. Later that afternoon, I followed Kathy, and we returned to our home.

During the drive home, I turned the volume up on the radio in my truck. A popular Christian song played. The singer sang about a day with no more tears, no more pain, and no more fears. I wondered if that was possible for Landon, or any of us again. Through watery eyes, I squinted to see the road ahead and the back of Kathy's car.

The next day, Landon slept. The antibiotic kicked in and fought the infection.

Thursday morning, Kathy drove back to the hospital in Winston-Salem, where, after receiving a clear blood culture test, the surgeon scheduled a 10:00 a.m. surgery to insert a new central line. I stayed in Sparta and worked.

Kathy called me when the nurses took Landon to the operating room. An urge to jump in my truck and drive to the hospital came over me, but I resisted. If I didn't work, we couldn't pay our bills or help Jeremiah and Shelly with theirs. I continued to work and waited for news.

After the surgeon placed a new line in Landon's left thigh, Kathy called and told me the surgery went well. She decided to stay the night at the hospital with Shelly and Landon so Jeremiah could go home and stay with the older boys.

A couple of hours later, Landon, awake and happy, played with his toys.

The surgeon didn't restart the TPN right away because the antibiotic in Landon's system was not compatible. Instead, he placed an anti-clotting solution in the line and prescribed a different antibiotic. To give the incompatible antibiotic time to clear Landon's body, he told Shelly not to restart the TPN until

9:00 p.m.

When the time came, Shelly attempted to flush the anti-clotting solution from the line, but it wouldn't budge. She tried to withdraw it and couldn't. The line was blocked. Shelly didn't know what else to do and told Kathy to call for a nurse.

A nurse came in and tried the same procedures without success. Sweat beads formed on her forehead while she struggled to unblock the new central line. The nurse pushed hard on the syringe plunger, and it gave way. A knot bulged on Landon's thigh. He screamed.

Kathy called me, crying. "The nurse busted the line. The surgeon might have to put a new one in."

I sat in a chair at the dining room table. Tears welled up. "Is he going to lose his second site?" I took a deep breath and held it.

"I don't know. The nurses called the surgeon. He scheduled an ultrasound for tomorrow morning to get a look at the line and see what happened." She sniffled.

I exhaled, hung up the phone, and laid my head on my arms on the table. This can't happen. He can't lose another access site so soon.

I couldn't stay away from the hospital any longer, so left for Winston-Salem the next morning and arrived at about the same time Jeremiah did. We met in the hall outside of Landon's room. My son's face was ashen white, his eyes circled by gray.

"Are you okay?" I asked.

"No, I didn't sleep much last night, my back hurts, the bills are piling up, and I'm worried about Landon."

I wanted to comfort my son but didn't know what to say. I placed my hand on his back in support as we entered Landon's room.

An hour later, an ultrasound confirmed what we feared, a ruptured line. The ultrasound also revealed the possibility of placing a new line a couple of inches up the vein, thus saving this access site. There was hope.

That afternoon, three days after losing the first central line, Landon lost his second line, but not his second access site. The surgeon managed to place a new line in the same vein just up an inch or so. We rejoiced because Landon still had four available access sites. The surgeon didn't want to take a chance on the line becoming blocked again, so before leaving the operating room, he started the TPN.

With the new line in place, the TPN flowed, and my anxiety eased. Still, we hadn't solved the problem with the adhesive bandages.

During the next couple of days, while Landon healed, the nurses experimented with different adhesive bandages, trying to find something that didn't cause an allergic reaction. They cut pieces from different types and brands of dressings and placed them on Landon's back. After several hours they removed the bandages. Landon had an allergic reaction to all but one, a film made with a latex-free adhesive. We wished we would have done this test before Landon's first central line became infected. The nurses sealed the site with this new bandage.

Sunday afternoon Kathy and I took the older brothers to the hospital for another visit. Landon now had bandages wrapped around both thighs; the one on the right covered the old access site that was healing nicely, and the one on the left protected the new site and central line. Shelly removed Landon from his crib and placed him in Roger's lap in the hospital reclining chair, then Ezekiel knelt on the floor beside his two brothers. Landon held the remote control and giggled. All three smiled while they watched cartoons together.

The next day, Monday, September 14, the surgeon discharged Landon from the hospital.

My little grandson suffered daily yet took everything in stride. His amazing spirit encouraged us. We had made big plans.

Now, it was time to launch those plans.

Chapter 18

Fundraising, Boston, and Holidays

There's something about a sick child that brings out the compassion in people. That's what we experienced with Landon. Some prayed, some donated money, and others gave their time and energy.

With the coin box campaign over, several times I met with people eager to plan more COTA fundraising events. I choked back tears each time I listened to a volunteer pitch an idea for a fundraiser, heard the passion in their voice, and saw the desire to help on their face.

Eager to raise money for Landon's transplant related expenses, I did everything I could to encourage and help them. In fall 2009, the fundraising campaign shifted into high gear.

Saturday, September 26, the Wings of Glory Christian Bikers Ministry held a "poker ride" for Landon. Motorcycle riders paid an entry fee to ride more than 150 miles through the Blue Ridge Mountains and collect a poker card from five different check-in stations. Despite the rainy day, about two dozen riders arrived, paid the fee, and roared out of the parking lot of a local store at 11:00 a.m.

The ride ended at 4:00 p.m. at the Pine Fork Baptist Church in Laurel Springs, North Carolina. Kathy and I watched the motorcycles thunder into the church parking lot. They compared their "poker hands" from the five cards they each collected along the route. The rider with the winning hand received half the entry fee money. The other half went to Landon. The crowd of rough, rowdy, wet bikers cheered when the winner stepped forward and donated the proceeds from his winning poker hand to Landon. A lump formed in my throat when the biker who stood beside me dabbed a tear from his eye.

After the ride, members of the church served hamburgers and hotdogs. A donation jar, at the end of the food line, soon filled with cash.

At 6:00 p.m., residents from the community gathered with the bikers for an auction of donated items and baked goods. Jeremiah, Shelly, and Landon arrived before the sale started. Five-month-old Landon sat on his mother's lap in the back of the room. Shelly took a spoon and smeared a little cake icing on his lips. He looked at a bearded biker, who came by to say hi, licked the icing from his lips, and smiled. I'm not sure if he smiled at the biker or because the icing tasted good.

The auctioneer's chant kept the excited crowd bidding fast

and furious.

I grabbed a piece of pie and a cup of coffee from the dessert table and sat beside a church member.

When the auctioneer held a big cake in the air, the church member leaned toward me and said, "That's sister Margaret's homemade walnut cake. You talk about good." He smacked his lips.

The auctioneer started the bid at twenty dollars. "Twenty now twenty-five, twenty-five now thirty, thirty now thirty-five."

At fifty dollars, it looked like the preacher had it. I almost choked on a mouthful of the pie when a big, whiskered biker in the back of the room shouted, "Fifty-five."

The auctioneer looked at the preacher. "Sixty?"

The preacher shook his head.

"What about fifty-six?"

The preacher nodded.

"Fifty-seven," the biker shouted.

The preacher lowered his eyes and shook his head.

The crowd cheered. The biker, who wore leather chaps and a leather vest, ran to the front of the room and claimed the cake. With a big smile, he held his prize in the air. The crowd cheered again.

I stood and clapped when he passed by me with the cake in his hands. He looked at me and winked. It was about Landon, not the cake. This biker might have looked rough on the outside, but he had a heart of gold on the inside. I couldn't figure out how he planned to get the cake home, in one piece, on his motorcycle.

After a fun day and evening, more than twelve hundred dollars went to Landon's COTA account. Every dollar raised got us a little closer to having the $75,000 for Landon's transplant.

Saturday, October 3, the Cracked Teapot—a small bistro on Main Street in Taylorsville, not far from where Jeremiah and Shelly lived—held a car show and a raffle. Kathy and I drove to Taylorsville to attend the fundraiser and support the volunteers who organized the event.

Owners of antique cars paid a fee to enter a vehicle in the show. The winners received a ribbon. The organizers donated the proceeds from the entry fees to Landon. During the car show, Kathy and I walked through the parking lot and admired the shiny vintage automobiles. We thanked the owners for participating and supporting our grandson.

Afterward, inside the Cracked Teapot, Landon and I sampled the ice cream. The business donated the day's receipts, as well as the proceeds from the raffle, to Landon's COTA account.

The next week I stared in awe at Landon's COTA webpage. A graphic of a thermometer indicated our progress toward the $75,000 goal. It registered more than ten percent, and volunteers planned for several more events in the coming weeks.

I felt good about the fundraising campaign, but I didn't feel good about Mom's situation. I worried about her.

My mother suffered from type-2 diabetes, and her doctor prescribed a daily insulin injection. Kathy went to Mom's apartment each morning to take her breakfast and give her the shot.

On a morning in mid-October, a couple of weeks before mom's seventy-sixth birthday, Kathy opened the door of my mother's apartment and found her on the floor between the sofa, where she slept most nights, and a coffee table. She had fallen sometime during the night and couldn't get up. Soaked with sweat, after thrashing around on the floor for hours and bruising her arms on the coffee table, she winced and cried when Kathy tried to help her. Kathy called for an ambulance.

At the hospital, the doctors didn't find a broken bone. Still, her shoulder hurt, and she couldn't move her arm. The doctors kept her in the hospital for three days, then transferred her to a rehabilitation center for in-house therapy. The employees at the center took good care of Mom, and I didn't worry as much about her. I concentrated more on Landon and upcoming fundraisers.

October 21, at a meeting of the New River Shrine Club in Sparta, the members presented me with a donation from the club and one from the Osborne Memorial Baptist Church.

With another scheduled trip to Boston coming up soon, which included an extended stay for testing, volunteers held one more fundraiser.

On the last Saturday in October, members of the Middle Cross Baptist Church in Pfafftown, North Carolina, about twelve miles northwest of Winston-Salem, held a rummage sale and donated the proceeds.

The fundraising events gave us the funds we needed to continue the fight for Landon's transplant.

On Monday, November 9, at 4:30 p.m., Jeremiah, Shelly, and Landon, again, boarded the Children's Flight of Hope aircraft at the airport in Statesville. The pilots flew them to Boston for the scheduled visit but didn't stay.

Three days later, with the tests done, the doctors discharged Landon. That same day a massive storm blew into New England. High winds buffeted the Boston area. When it became apparent the pilots couldn't return, the Children's Flight of Hope bought Jeremiah, Shelly, and Landon tickets to fly home on a commercial flight. "Oh no," I thought, not another commercial flight. But we didn't have much choice. At least the flight was with a major airline, not a cut-rate carrier. Saturday, they flew home without any problems.

We didn't plan any fundraising events for the last two months of the year. We hoped to spend a quiet holiday season with our family. But it didn't start that way. Three days before Thanksgiving, Jeremiah almost got arrested.

The skin around Landon's central line became red, and a lump formed in his thigh.

Fearing a blood clot, ruptured line, or an infection, Jeremiah and Shelly rushed Landon to the emergency room, where the ER physician took one look at Landon's central line and said he was going to remove it.

Jeremiah jumped between the doctor and his son. His face

blushed red, and he raised his voice. "Oh, hell no, you're not."

Jeremiah knew what needed to happen and how precious the central line was. The ER doctor didn't and wouldn't listen to reason. The doctor called for security and threatened to have Jeremiah arrested.

The security officer restrained Jeremiah. Shelly wrapped her arms around her son and demanded to speak to the emergency room supervisor. Tears flowed while she convinced the supervisor to call Landon's surgeon before they hauled Jeremiah off to jail or did anything else.

When they got Landon's surgeon on the phone, he told the ER doctor to leave the central line alone and admit Landon to the hospital. He did, and they didn't take Jeremiah to jail.

After that incident, Landon's surgeon told Jeremiah and Shelly to call him before taking Landon to the emergency room. He would pre-admit Landon to the hospital and bypass the ER.

The next morning an ultrasound and lab cultures revealed a site infection and not a blood clot, a ruptured line, or a line infection. With no need to remove the central line, the surgeon started antibiotics.

The antibiotic worked. Thanksgiving Day, with Roger and Ezekiel at our home, Kathy and I prepared a big meal. We expected the doctor to discharge Landon from the hospital, and that he and his parents would join us for an afternoon meal. But a last-minute blood test revealed his hemoglobin was low. The doctor ordered an iron infusion, which required them to remain at the hospital most of the day. They finally joined us for a late evening meal.

Before we ate, we gathered around our old farmhouse table, held hands, and gave thanks for the life of seven-month-old Landon.

Friday, December 4, three motorcycle enthusiasts from the American Legion Post in Mount Airy, North Carolina, surprised me when they stopped by our business and presented me with a donation. Landon's story continued to spread amongst the motorcycle community. This group wanted to help.

In early December, the rehabilitation center decided they couldn't do anything else for Mom. She would need to go home or to a longer-term facility. We didn't think we could take care of her at home, so they transferred her to a rest home in a neighboring town, about ten miles away. Not far, but too far for us to visit more than once a day. That didn't make Mom happy.

During December, one day each week, Jeremiah and Shelly took Landon back to the hospital in Winston-Salem for iron infusions. The doctors treated him in outpatient, but the trip and the procedure took most of a day. On the infusion days, Kathy took a day off work and drove to our son's home to meet Ezekiel and Roger after school. A couple of times, she spent the night at Jeremiah's house, slept on the sofa, and drove home the next day.

The time we took off work to help with Landon made a negative impact on our finances. Jeremiah managed to work a little and complete a few projects. Shelly picked up a part-time job as a waitress at a local restaurant. Still, for us to keep our household bills paid and help Jeremiah and Shelly with theirs took most of what Kathy and I earned. We didn't have much money to spend on Christmas gifts. We didn't care that we couldn't buy a lot, so long as we could buy a little something for each of our five grandsons and spend time with them.

Five days before Christmas, a snowstorm blanketed the area. Almost ten inches of snow fell at Jeremiah and Shelly's home, more than thirteen inches at our home in the mountains. The temperatures plummeted into the low teens. For several days we didn't venture out on the treacherous roads unless we were in my four-wheel-drive truck.

The day before Christmas, members of a church in Taylorsville surprised Jeremiah, Shelly, and the boys when they made their way up the family's long snow-covered driveway with a box of food for a Christmas meal and a box of gifts for the family. Shelly said it really felt like Christmas when the group stood in the front yard, sang a Christmas carol, and then prayed for their family, Landon, in particular.

At our home, Kathy wrapped Christmas presents, baked cookies, and fretted about the icy roads. She feared it wouldn't be safe for us to travel to Jeremiah's house, and we would miss Landon's first Christmas.

Christmas Eve, I drove to the rest home and took my mother Christmas gifts—two skeins of yarn and a box of cookies. Mom was happy to see me and eager for some company. I stayed late, and we talked about Landon while she crocheted.

The next morning, Kathy and I traveled to Jeremiah and Shelly's house. A few slick spots kept me alert and Kathy on edge.

We arrived safely at a little before 9:00 a.m. I carried a box of gifts wrapped in colorful Christmas paper from our car and placed them under the tree.

Landon also sat under the Christmas tree. He wore a tee-shirt, diaper, and a red and white Santa toboggan. A stainless-steel pole beside the Christmas tree held his TPN pump, and a long clear plastic tube connected the pump to Landon's central line. A knitted gauze stocking covered his left leg and protected the line and access site. His eyes twinkled when Kathy sat in a chair beside him. Ezekiel read the name tags on the presents and handed them out.

Landon, having already opened presents from Santa earlier that morning, knew what to do. He tore into the paper and squealed. We laughed. Jeremiah followed behind his son and held the central line so it wouldn't get snagged. The toys didn't interest Landon until he unwrapped, or helped unwrap, all the gifts. Then, he sat on the floor surrounded by stuffed animals and piles of torn, crumpled wrapping paper.

Two hours later, Jeremiah dressed Landon in a snug, warm snowsuit. He carried him to the yard where the three of us watched Ezekiel slide on a snow-covered hill with a new sled he had received as a gift. Roger, in his bedroom, strummed a tune on his new electric guitar. In the kitchen, Kathy and Shelly cooked.

That evening, after a lovely Christmas dinner, Jeremiah and Shelly cleaned the kitchen while Kathy and I sat with Landon on the sofa.

"Landon wants to show you something," Kathy said. She

looked at Landon. "Show Papaw your teefies." She pointed at her mouth and grinned.

Landon looked at me, smiled, and revealed two little bottom teeth.

I smiled back.

"He's gained two more pounds," Kathy boasted.

Other than Landon's pale white face, which made the red tint in his hair even more apparent, he looked like an average eight-month-old child, even a little chubby.

I gazed into my grandson's ocean-blue eyes and felt a connection. I knew he couldn't understand what happened to him and why he suffered. Yet, his eyes told me that his spirit did, why he had to fight for his life—every day. His eyes beckoned me to continue the fight with him.

Landon looked at his grandmother's face, then laid his head on her breast and closed his eyes. I closed mine and leaned my head back on the sofa.

The furnace kicked on. The scent of the Christmas tree wafted on the warm air and filled the room with the smell of pine, a Christmas smell. Soft guitar music echoed from Roger's bedroom. Kathy and Landon dozed, so did I.

Chapter 19

Losing More Lines

Landon's central line broke.

"No, not another central line," I cried out to God when I heard the news.

Jeremiah and Shelly did everything they could to prevent a break. But, with an active eight-and-a-half-month-old who crawled and explored, it happened fast and took us by surprise. The line didn't break entirely in two. That could have caused Landon to bleed out—something Jeremiah says gave him nightmares. The line kinked and cracked about an inch above the skin.

Sunday evening, January 10, 2010, almost four months to the day after the surgeon placed the third central line, Jeremiah called and told the surgeon what happened.

"Get Landon to the hospital," the surgeon said. "The line

might be salvageable." He instructed Jeremiah on how to clamp the line so Landon wouldn't bleed, or bacteria wouldn't enter the line.

Jeremiah called and told us what happened. Kathy packed a bag and left for Jeremiah's house to stay with Roger and Ezekiel.

After she did, I couldn't sleep, so I wrote a post for Landon's blog, asked for prayers, and waited to find out what would happen.

At the hospital, Jeremiah and Shelly held their son as still as possible for more than an hour while a technician tried to splice the line. Landon squirmed and cried.

A little before 3:00 a.m., I sat at our dining table and sipped warm coffee. The phone rang.

Jeremiah sobbed. "They couldn't fix the line."

I closed my eyes, lowered my head, and listened.

He then said, "The surgeon will remove it and place another line in a different access site this afternoon. I'm afraid he's going to run out of sites before he can get a transplant."

I sensed the fear in my son's voice. "He'll make it," I said, trying to comfort him. "After the surgeon places the new line, Landon will still have three unused access sites. He'll make it." I tried to sound confident, but I wasn't.

In the morning, disappointed and tired, I went to our shop and worked. I struggled to concentrate while I stapled new upholstery fabric to an old club chair with a pneumatic stapler and did the math in my head. It didn't add up. If Landon continued to lose lines every three to four months, he would run out of sites before he could get a transplant, and that's if an infection didn't kill him first. The negative thoughts flooded my mind. Through tear-filled eyes, I looked at my work and pulled the trigger. The staple gun drove a one-half inch staple into my left index finger. In my career, as an upholsterer, I've stapled my fingers several dozen times. To accidentally staple a finger now and then is an occupational hazard, it hurts, but it happens. This time it hurt more than most. I grabbed a pair of pliers and pulled the staple from the bone. With my right hand, I clutched my finger and squeezed. For several minutes, I held my breath, clenched my teeth, and let the tears flow—tears for my throbbing finger that turned into tears for Landon.

At noon, I closed the shop and drove to the hospital in Winston-Salem. Not to have my finger looked at but for Landon's surgery. I couldn't stay away. I wanted to hold my wife and watch what happened to my grandson.

After she got the older boys off to school, Kathy drove to the hospital, where I met her in the hall outside of our grandson's room and showed her my swollen finger. She kissed it.

"I'm sorry," she said, "but, Jeremiah and Shelly are taking this hard. Let's try to keep Landon happy until time for the surgery."

We suppressed the pain we both felt, smiled, entered the room, and played with our grandson like nothing was wrong.

That afternoon, the surgeon removed the central line from Landon's thigh and placed a new line in a vein on the right side of his chest. To protect the line from germs and Landon's little fingers, the surgeon bandaged the site with a square of adhesive film, the one that didn't make Landon's skin turn red. The surgeon addressed another problem.

Landon had outgrown the G-tube—the medical device in his belly used to pump formula into his stomach. The surgeon had taught Jeremiah how to reinsert the G-tube if it ever popped out. It did, several times. Also, a rash had developed around the tube. The surgeon replaced it with a larger one, then treated the infected skin with an antibiotic cream.

A couple of hours after the surgery, back in his hospital room, Landon woke, sat in his bed, and looked at the new tubes, wires, and bandages. The corners of his mouth turned down. His eyes drooped, and tears formed. He wasn't happy because the lines wouldn't allow him to stand in his crib, move about, and play.

Shelly looked at her son's sad face, wiped away her tears, then wrapped her arms around Landon and hugged him.

Kathy's chin quivered. She showed Landon a new helium-filled balloon she bought at the hospital gift shop and forced a smile. He reached for it.

Before Landon woke, Shelly had wrapped a disposable diaper around her son's right hand to protect an IV in his hand. The diaper looked like a white boxing glove. She helped Landon stand in his crib and checked to make sure the lines weren't tangled or snagged.

Kathy held the balloon in front of Landon and showed him how to punch it with his diaper-covered hand. Soon the tears disappeared. He laughed and giggled each time he smacked the balloon.

Jeremiah hadn't said much all day. He sat in a chair, watched his mother play with his son, and didn't smile.

I pulled a chair over and sat beside him. I knew what his thoughts were. "Jeremiah, this is not your fault."

He closed his eyes and lowered his head. His drooping shoulders carried an invisible burden. I tried to think of something more to say, words to lighten his load. I couldn't. But I sat beside my son and felt his pain.

Two days later, Landon went home. With the IV lines gone, Jeremiah and Shelly cycled the TPN and the formula. They kept the tubes untangled so their son could crawl and explore. At times, learning to walk, Landon pushed himself around the room in a round plastic walker. Shelly kept him corralled in the living room. Having him home, not in the hospital, made us happy. It didn't last long.

Six days later, after a long Martin Luther King Jr. holiday weekend, Landon got sick. Shelly sent Roger and Ezekiel to the school bus stop then went to Landon's crib to wake him. She found him lethargic and hot. Alarmed, she called for Jeremiah. Together they checked his temperature—103 degrees. Now in emergency mode, they called Landon's surgeon, told him about the fever, and sped out of the driveway and back to the hospital.

There, a recheck of Landon's temperature registered 104. The nurses worked fast. They hung two bags of antibiotics and connected them to an IV drip, then placed ice packs around Landon's body.

Kathy and I rushed to the hospital and arrived at about noon. The looks on the faces of our son and daughter-in-law alarmed us. Jeremiah and Shelly sat on opposite sides of Landon's bed and wiped his face, head, and body with a wet washcloth. We stood beside Shelly and looked at our grandson. He slept but thrashed when one of his parents touched him with a damp cloth.

"His temperature is down a little, 102.2," Jeremiah said. "When we stop rubbing him with a damp cloth, his temperature rises."

Kathy placed the palm of her hand on Landon's forehead. She stroked the wet red curls matted to his head, took the cloth from Jeremiah's hand, and placed it on her grandson's head.

A few minutes after Kathy and I arrived, Landon's surgeon walked into the room. He didn't smile, and he didn't sugar coat his words. "I think Landon has a line infection and line infections kill."

Confused, I asked, "Is this not like the other infections?"

"No, those were site infections in the skin around the central line. This time bacteria entered Landon's bloodstream. If we don't knock it out soon, he'll lose this central line, or worse."

I understood "worse" meant my grandson would die. "What can we do?"

The surgeon reached for the bag of fluids hanging from the metal pole beside of Landon's bed and read the label. "We are giving him a powerful antibiotic. We've drawn blood for cultures. When the lab tells us what we are dealing with, we'll know better how to fight it. Until then, keep him cool." The surgeon rubbed the back of his hand across Landon's cheek, then left the room.

I hadn't seen my grandson this sick since his birth. I wanted to help him and did the only thing I knew to do. I took the cloth from my daughter-in-law's hand and placed it on Landon's neck. He squirmed but didn't wake. I looked at his red face and felt the damp sheets around his body.

We stayed in the quiet, dim room through the next day. Jeremiah, Shelly, Kathy, and I took turns, wiped Landon with wet cloths, and watched the antibiotics drip into the IV line. We didn't pray aloud, but we prayed.

The next morning, the lab gave us a name for the enemy, methicillin-susceptible staphylococcus aureus (MSSA). MSSA causes skin infections and likely caused the earlier infections around Landon's central line. It possibly entered Landon's bloodstream when his central line broke, weeks earlier. The bacteria had colonized and now attacked his body. The good news was, as the name implies, this bug is susceptible to antibiotics.

At 6:00 p.m., almost thirty-six hours after Shelly discovered her sick child, the fever broke. Jeremiah and Shelly, relieved, collapsed into the recliners in Landon's hospital room. Landon slept. Kathy and I, exhausted, drove home.

The next morning, better rested, I drove to the rest home to visit Mom.

I eased the door open to the dim room. Mom sat in a rocking chair with her tattered Bible in her lap. She smiled, and I sat on the bed beside her. On her dresser were pictures of me, my sister, my brother, and our families. She didn't say anything about Kathy and me not visiting for the past few days but pointed at the pictures.

"I have three children and nine grandchildren," she said.

"Yes, Mom. You do."

With some difficulty—I didn't correct her or help—she recited each of our names.

"And I have great-grandchildren." Again, she recited the names. When she came to Landon, she said, "I held that sweet baby when he was born, and the doctor said he was going to die. Didn't I?" A tear dropped from her cheek.

"Yes, you did." A vision of my mother holding newborn Landon popped into my mind. My throat tightened, and I swallowed hard.

"He didn't die, did he?"

"No, he didn't. He's been sick, but he didn't die."

She held her Bible with both hands. "There's no need to worry. I've been praying for him. He's okay, isn't he?"

"Yes, he's okay." But I wasn't so sure. If only I had the kind of faith my mom did. I stood to leave.

"I have three children and nine grandchildren, don't I?"

"Yes, you do, Mom."

I pulled the door closed behind me as she recited our names.

The next day, with the fever gone, Landon played in his

hospital bed. Both parents watched and kept their son from getting tangled in his lines. He felt better, but he couldn't go home until he finished a round of the powerful antibiotics. MSSA can hide in the body. A few days or weeks later, when the doctors think they have defeated the bacteria, the bug can re-emerge and make him sick again. The longer Landon could remain on the antibiotics, the better.

On the afternoon of January 25, after a week in the hospital, Jeremiah and Shelly brought Landon home. Their family reunited and soon settled into a routine again.

The battle with the bacteria caused Landon to lose three pounds. He gained it back during the cold, snowy February. Then came March and more central line problems.

On the first day of the month, Landon's central line snagged on his toe. When he kicked, the line pulled out. The line didn't pull out of his chest, but the cuff came through the skin. It wasn't secure. Again, we couldn't blame anyone. What could Jeremiah and Shelly have done? Tied Landon to a bed and not let him move until he got a transplant?

At the hospital, the surgeon determined he couldn't put the line back in.

March 2, Landon lost the line and his third access site. The surgeon placed a new line in a vein on the other side of Landon's chest and sent him home that evening. The pulled line and the surgery to replace it happened fast. We didn't have much time to worry, mourn, or grieve about the lost line. I do remember the feeling of helplessness.

Would my ten-month-old grandson run out of sites before he grew big enough for a transplant? The thoughts made me sick, so I chose to focus on the positive and making good memories while we could.

Saturday, March 13, Jeremiah and Shelly brought their sons to Sparta to attend the annual Cub Scout Pinewood Derby.

Days and weeks before the race, adults—fathers, grandfathers, mentors, etc.—helped Cub Scouts carve model cars from blocks of wood, paint the cars, and place axles and little plastic wheels on them. Jeremiah, an Eagle Scout who had built several pinewood derby cars when he was a Cub Scout, helped Ezekiel build a car. I helped my other grandson, Gavin, make one.

At the derby, Ezekiel placed his car at the starting line on the high end of the wood track. He shook hands with his competitor, a fellow Cub Scout. The track official, an assistant Scoutmaster, pressed a button and released the cars. The crowd cheered.

On this rare day in public, dressed in a blue sweatsuit with a grey hoodie, Landon, almost eleven-months-old, tottled around the arena with the help of his aunt Jessica. He sucked on his orange pacifier and made new friends. He jumped, squealed, and mimicked the excitement of the scouts when the cars zoomed down the track. Lights flashed for the winner, and Ezekiel did a victory dance.

The crowd cheered louder; so did Landon. I smiled as I watched my grandsons having fun.

That pinewood derby was the last scouting event I presided

over. Twenty-five years after becoming a Scout leader, I surrendered the Cubmaster position to another leader. I needed to focus on our business and helping with Landon.

I thought about our experience with Landon's transplant journey. What a rollercoaster of emotional highs and lows. I wondered what could be next.

Chapter 20

Duke

We thought Boston was the best place for Landon's transplant, but insurance had other ideas. Not only were we fighting to keep Landon alive, but we were also gearing up to again do battle with Medicaid.

Again, God had other plans.

"Are you sitting?" Jeremiah said when I answered the phone. "If not, you should. You're not going to believe this. Duke University Medical Center has established a pediatric intestinal transplant team, and they want Landon as one of their first patients."

My knees wobbled, and I eased into a chair. "Did you say, Duke? The Duke, in Durham, North Carolina?"

"Yes, Dad. The Duke. Two-and-one-half-hours away. They want Landon."

I leaned back, closed my eyes, and swallowed hard. In my mind, God brought together a dream team of intestinal transplant surgeons and established the transplant program at Duke just for Landon.

In early 2010, while the Duke team worked to prepare the transition, the doctors in Boston made decisions and recommendations about Landon's TPN formula and nutrition. Landon's original surgeon, in Winston-Salem, managed the central line and treated infections.

In late March, another infection caused Landon's temperature to rise to 101. Irritable but coherent, he whined and cried while his parents rushed him to the hospital in Winston-Salem. There, a nurse initiated a familiar routine; she drew blood for testing and administered antibiotics.

Kathy and I arrived at the hospital in time to hear the lab report.

"Gram-positive cocci," the surgeon said. "A nasty bug, and dangerous when it's in the bloodstream. We'll watch it close, but it should respond to the antibiotics."

Like the last infection, caused by a different bacterium, this one must have entered through the central line. I wondered how this could happen since Jeremiah and Shelly were careful about sanitation around Landon.

Because Landon was not as sick as he had been in February, Shelly remained with her son at the hospital while Jeremiah went home to care for Roger and Ezekiel, and to work. Kathy and I went home also.

Three days passed.

The antibiotic worked, Landon's fever broke, and the surgeon discharged him.

Shelly and Landon returned home, where Jeremiah tended to Landon, and Shelly recovered. The next morning, rested, Shelly prepared for Ezekiel's ninth birthday party that afternoon, which that year also happened to be Good Friday.

April is a month of birthdays for Jeremiah and Shelly's family, beginning with Ezekiel's. Shelly planned a late afternoon get together to celebrate, and Kathy and I wanted to be there.

Before we left, I visited Mom at the rest home and met with the chief financial officer who had called the day before.

The financial officer looked across her cluttered desk and said, "I'm sorry, but your mother's insurance will not pay for her to remain here much longer."

Three months earlier, the rest home admitted Mom for continued physical therapy, not indefinite convalescence. We knew the arrangement wouldn't last and continued to pay the rent on Mom's apartment. We hoped she would get better and return home. But she couldn't, not without someone there to give her full-time care. We couldn't afford to pay for in-home care any more than we could afford to pay for her to remain at the rest home.

"Can you do anything?" I pleaded.

With her elbows on the desk and her fingertips together

touching her chin as if praying, she exhaled, then I learned that Mom fell beside her bed the day before. She bruised her hip on the floor, her shin on a chair, and now used a walker to steady herself.

"Since your mother fell and is having problems walking, we can begin therapy with the hope she will recover. I can get her an extension for a few more months, but after that, you'll need to make other arrangements."

Knowing she might have bent the rules a little to help us, I shook the woman's hand and thanked her.

I still didn't know what we would do. But whew, at least the financial officer gave us a few months to figure it out.

After the visit, during the drive to Taylorsville, Kathy gazed out the passenger window and, in a somber voice, said, "Ezekiel didn't play football last fall. He's not trying out for soccer this spring. He's missing out on a lot, and I loved watching him play."

"Jeremiah and Shelly are focused on taking care of Landon," I said. "They don't have time to take Zeke to practice, and they don't have money for registrations and equipment. It's the best they can do."

Young Ezekiel understood and didn't ask for much. He went to school and visited Landon during the frequent hospital stays. Other than that, Ezekiel rarely left home. Once outgoing, he now stayed in his room and played video games most of the time.

For a few moments, I thought about my grandson's situation and how his life had changed since the birth of his little brother, almost a year earlier. My throat tightened. "Let's invite him to come home with us this evening. He can use his new fishing rod tomorrow morning." I looked in the rearview mirror at the fishing pole wrapped in birthday paper in the back seat and smiled. Kathy wiped a tear from her cheek and nodded.

The next morning, I rose an hour before daybreak and fixed a breakfast of sausage, eggs, and biscuits for Ezekiel and me before we headed to the mountain stream behind our house. I knew this stream well and took us to a spot where we should have success right away.

On the bank, I pointed across the water to the first hole. "Do you see that dark water under the tree limb?"

Ezekiel stood beside me and acknowledged that he did.

"Cast your hook into the dark water."

The evening before, Ezekiel had practiced casting in our backyard. Now skilled, he made a perfect cast to the fishing hole. The size six hook, with two kernels of yellow corn on it, landed in the center of the dark pool with a plop. The water swirled. My grandson jerked the pole and reeled in the eighteen-inch rainbow trout.

"Good job, Zeke," I said, slapping my grandson on the back. "Let me get a picture." Ezekiel struggled and held the fish with both hands. He laughed. The camera clicked, and I smiled.

The next afternoon, Easter, Kathy and I took Ezekiel home and stayed for several hours to visit with Landon. A little unsteady but now walking, Landon, barefoot, wore a yellow onesie and his red backpack with the TPN and pumps inside. Kathy held his hand while he explored the backyard. His delicate red curls fluttered in the warm breeze.

Sixteen days later, on Landon's birthday, Kathy called and asked Shelly to hold the phone to Landon's ear. Kathy and I sang, "Happy birthday."

"He's smiling," Shelly said.

The rest of the day, at work, Kathy and I talked about Landon's first year.

"Look at all he's been through," I said, "the surgeries, the central lines, the trips to Boston, the infections, and he's still with us, still fighting. God put people in Landon's life to help him." I pulled a tissue from the box on the desk and handed it to Kathy.

"I thank God for Landon every day." She dabbed her eyes with the tissue.

With both hands on the table of Kathy's sewing machine, I leaned forward until my face was close to hers. "God placed Landon in a strong family and gave him a loving grandmother." I kissed her.

Two days later, April 22, 2010, Jeremiah, Shelly, Landon, and I met with another group of people that God placed in Landon's life, the transplant team at Duke.

Excited to meet the team we had read about on the Internet, we waited in a quiet exam room. Landon sat on the exam table with a green pacifier in his mouth.

The door opened. Four doctors, in white lab coats, entered

the exam room, followed by a man about thirty-years-old who wore khakis, a light blue shirt, and a tie. A doctor with short blond hair introduced herself as the transplant team leader. From our research, we knew what she had accomplished. A pioneer in pediatric intestinal transplants, she looked younger than I had imagined.

She smiled at Landon, ran her fingers through his hair, and touched his nose with the tip of her index finger. Landon pulled his pacifier from his mouth and smiled at the doctor.

Another young female doctor with shoulder-length brown curly hair stood beside the team leader. She introduced herself as an assistant and another transplant surgeon. The two male doctors were assistants as well.

The team leader pointed to the man in khakis. "He is the transplant coordinator, your contact person. He'll schedule your visits, answer questions, and help with anything you need." She turned her attention back to Landon. "He looks good. I'm sure you know that most babies born with his condition don't survive. Those that do soon develop liver failure. How did you get him to a year old, looking this good, and relatively healthy?" She waved her hand over Landon.

In less than ten minutes, Jeremiah, Shelly, and I recapped everything that our family and the doctors had done to save Landon's liver and keep him healthy during his first year.

Jeremiah said, "Our goal is to get Landon a transplant while he's still strong enough to survive."

With the other doctors nodding, the team leader smiled and looked at Landon. "It's worked so far."

I looked at the team leader and then scanned the eyes of the other doctors. "The surgeon in Winston-Salem saved Landon's life soon after his birth, and we give the doctors in Boston credit for saving Landon's liver, but where do we go from here? What can you do for my grandson?"

"We've studied Landon's records." Again, the other doctors nodded while the team leader spoke. "We want to do more tests to look at what has happened in the past few months. After we evaluate the results, we'll make a plan."

As the meeting came to an end, the team leader again ran her fingers through Landon's hair and smiled.

With the pacifier still in his mouth, Landon gave her a big grin and followed the surgeon with his eyes.

She wiggled her fingers at him while she exited the room with the other doctors.

The coordinator stayed with Jeremiah and Shelly to schedule an admission date for Landon. I entertained my grandson and discreetly wiped tears until they finished.

Outside, I took a deep breath. In front of Duke University Medical Center, with the Carolina-blue sky in the background, I snapped a picture of Jeremiah, Shelly, and Landon. A copy of the photo hangs above my desk, where I wrote this book.

This hospital and the team would give my grandson a second chance at a long life. I felt it deep inside. The looks on the faces of

Jeremiah, Shelly, and even Landon, told me they felt it too.

We headed home to celebrate Landon's second chance and to kick off his second year of life with a big party, knowing the roller coaster ride continued.

Chapter 21

Birthday, Infections, and Landon Visits

At his first birthday party, April 25, 2010, Landon was king for a day.

About a dozen of Landon's young cousins and friends gathered around him. Kathy placed a gold paper crown on his head. She extended both hands, palms up, toward Landon and said, "King Landon." The children jumped, squealed, and clapped. An equal number of adults applauded.

Aware of the many threats that could cut Landon's life short, I wanted to document the milestone. I stood on the periphery of the group and snapped pictures. At least we would have photos of Landon's first birthday party. I swallowed hard and wondered if he would survive to celebrate a second.

Shelly shouted to the children, "Go play." The excited young partygoers fanned out from the pavilion and ran toward the playground equipment where they laughed, climbed, and swung.

From his perch on the picnic table, Landon watched the children play then held his hands out to his grandmother. He wanted to join the children. He wanted to play.

Kathy removed him from the table, stood him on the ground, and held his hand. Wearing a green long-sleeved shirt, blue denim pants, and his gold crown, he waddled toward a slide. I followed behind with a packet of sanitary wipes.

I wiped the five-foot-high slide, then sat Landon on top. He grabbed my arm and tensed.

Kathy, on the opposite side of the slide, held his other hand. I looked at my wife while she looked at our grandson. She smiled. Her eyes gleamed. In a soft voice, she said to Landon, "We've got you."

At the pavilion, Shelly rushed around four wood picnic tables and placed party settings. She turned toward the playground and shouted to the children, "Let's cut the cake."

After a second, then a third call, followed by a little coaxing from parents, the children ran toward the pavilion. With help from Kathy and me, Landon followed.

His expression turned to confusion when the children sang, "Happy birthday." Then, seated on Roger's lap, and with the help of his two big brothers, he puffed at the flame and blew out the candle on the cake. We clapped and cheered.

Jeremiah watched from outside the pavilion with three other young fathers. They talked and laughed. I hadn't seen my son relax with friends in more than a year.

As Landon opened his presents, I hoped the good times would continue. They didn't.

Two days after the birthday party, Shelly and Jeremiah rushed Landon back to the hospital in Winston-Salem with another high fever—103. A lab test revealed that the same bacteria which caused the last infection also caused this one. The bacteria had hidden in Landon's body and reemerged.

The surgeon suggested that it possibly hid in the central line. I hung my head. He can't lose another central line.

With the process of transferring Landon's care to Duke almost complete, the doctors in Winston-Salem informed Duke about this illness. Duke recommended the use of ethanol in the central line instead of the blood thinner. The ethanol would not only prevent a blood clot but could kill the bacteria in the line.

The combination of antibiotics and ethanol worked. Six days later, with the fever gone and Landon feeling better, Jeremiah and Shelly brought him home. They also brought ethanol with them and continued using it in the central line.

But, the next day, the line blocked. They didn't take Landon back to Winston-Salem but chose to drive the extra hour and a half to Duke. A nurse there, experienced at using ethanol in central lines, unblocked the line and removed the blood clot. Then, before they left the hospital, the nurse instructed Jeremiah and Shelly on how to use the ethanol to prevent another blood clot.

Sixteen days later, Jeremiah, Shelly, and Landon returned to

Durham for a scheduled day of tests. After a long day at Duke, where they poked, prodded, and scanned Landon, he and his parents returned home with good news and bad news.

First, the good news. Landon's central line looked good. The doctors believed the antibiotics and the ethanol had killed the bacteria. But the bad news made our hearts sink. Inflamed ducts in Landon's liver and an enlarged spleen indicated damage caused by the TPN. Also, Landon had lost weight. The transplant coordinator scheduled another appointment at Duke in a month for a liver biopsy and a meeting with the transplant doctor. She wanted to discuss the test results and a plan.

I shook my head. What plan? We had a plan. Get Landon to twenty pounds or two years old, strong enough to survive a transplant, and raise enough money to cover our family's transplant-related expenses.

We hoped that not traveling to Boston or another distant city for Landon's medical care or his transplant would reduce the amount of money we needed to raise. But we didn't know what the future held and kept our fundraising goal at $75,000.

In late May, the Marvin United Methodist Church held another fundraiser. The church, located in Stony Point, North Carolina, about twelve miles west of Statesville, is the home church of Shelly's maternal grandfather's family. The members scheduled the hamburger and hot dog fundraiser to take place from noon until 6:00 p.m. Participants could eat lunch or supper, or both meals at the church, for a donation.

When we arrived, a lady who sat at one of the dining tables

pointed at Landon, in Shelly's arms, and said, "There he is."

The other diners applauded.

A man, who I later learned was Shelly's great uncle, raised his hand and said, "Praise God."

Shelly held Landon's arm and helped him wave to the crowd.

Through misty eyes, I nodded and acknowledged the reception for my grandson.

We entered the fellowship hall, where people stood in a line for food. Workers prepared and packed carry-out meals in large Styrofoam coolers.

A man sat at a small table by the door and collected donations.

I asked him, "Where are all those carry-out meals going?"

"We have an order for almost two hundred meals at a factory a few miles from here," he said.

During the afternoon, people joined in a cakewalk on the church lawn. Thirty to forty participants paid a dollar each, formed a circle, and walked while a band played.

Kathy held Landon and walked several times. She handed him off to Shelly, who danced around the circle. Shelly smiled and laughed, but dark rings surrounded her eyes.

Jeremiah and I sat under a shade tree and watched the activities. My son yawned a couple of times, then closed his eyes and dozed.

On that single day in May 2010, the Marvin United Methodist Church raised $4,360.00 for Landon and pushed the total donated past the $20,000 mark.

With big smiles on our faces, Kathy and I left. We drove toward home while the radio blared an upbeat Christian song. We celebrated. But the faces of my son and daughter-in-law flashed in my mind. My heart grew heavy.

I lowered the volume on the radio. "Did you notice how tired Jeremiah and Shelly looked and acted?"

"Yes, they need a break." Kathy closed her eyes and leaned her head back on the headrest.

I thought for a moment, then said, "Why don't we invite them to come to our house for a weekend?"

My wife raised her head and smiled. "We can watch Landon while they go out for the night."

Kathy longed to have Landon spend a night with us. Each of our other grandsons spent a night with us when they were infants. She missed that with Landon.

Outside of a hospital, no one other than Jeremiah or Shelly had taken care of fourteen-month-old Landon through an entire night. Way past time for the parents to take a break. The next day, Kathy called and gave the invitation.

Two weekends later, Kathy stood at the window and looked out at our long gravel driveway. "They should be here any minute. I'm scared. What if something bad happens to Landon while we are taking care of him?"

"Relax," I said. "Jeremiah and Shelly won't be too far away."

A few minutes later, they arrived. Kathy rushed to the car to help Shelly with Landon. I helped Jeremiah unload the luggage.

In the house, I unpacked Landon's medical supplies and pumps while Jeremiah placed a couple of bags of TPN and formula in the refrigerator.

At our dining room table, Shelly pulled a notebook from the luggage. The journal contained pages of handwritten notes, schedules, and a list of medicines. She reviewed the instructions with Kathy.

In our living room, I watched Jeremiah connect a bag of TPN to Landon's central line and turn on the pumps. "He'll be good through the night," Jeremiah said.

"Where's the pole for the pumps and TPN bags?" I said.

"He doesn't need the pole." Jeremiah reached for a black bag that looked like a computer bag with wheels on it. "I made this."

My son unzipped the bag and revealed a thin piece of plywood cut to fit in the bottom of the bag where a computer would have been. He had screwed four casters through the bag and into the plywood so it would roll on the floor. Jeremiah placed the two battery-operated pumps, a bag of TPN, and a bag of lipids in the modified computer bag. A perfect fit. He zipped the bag shut but left enough room for the five-foot line that connected to the central line in Landon's chest. A shorter, four-foot shoestring, tied to the bag and then to Landon's clothes, allowed him to pull the bag without pulling on the lines.

"Ingenious," I said. "You need to patent this." I smiled.

Jeremiah reminded me of my father. He could fix anything.

"First," Kathy said, "you two need to get out of here." She waved the back of her hand toward Jeremiah and Shelly. "We can handle Landon. Go." Her eyes gleamed.

If the unexpected happened, our son and daughter-in-law wouldn't be far away. They decided to go to a restaurant, then to a movie at the closest theater to our home, thirty miles away, and then return here to sleep in our spare bedroom. Landon would sleep in a portable crib in our room where we could tend to him.

Kathy held Landon.

Shelly kissed him on both cheeks and then on his forehead. Tears filled her eyes. I wondered if she had second thoughts about leaving.

Jeremiah put an arm around his wife. "Come on, Shelly. We'll be late for the movie." He smiled, but tears formed in his eyes also.

"You two go and have a good time. We'll call if we need you," I said in the most reassuring voice I could muster.

Kathy and I stood on the front porch with Landon and waved. The car rolled out the driveway. From the open passenger window, Shelly shouted instructions until they were out of hearing distance.

I looked at Kathy. "What do we do now?"

"Let's play." She emphasized the word "play."

In the house, Kathy placed Landon on the living room floor. He waddled from the sofa to a chair. Then to the dining room and the kitchen. The black bag rolled behind him.

For a couple of hours, Kathy and I chased Landon around our home. And sometimes, he pursued us. We laughed. He giggled. A few times, the bag got hooked on a chair or table. I rushed and dislodged it. We played until bedtime, and the three of us grew tired.

Kathy placed Landon in his crib. I helped her prepare him for the night. We connected a tube that carried nutritional formula to the G-tube and into his stomach and started the pump. It didn't take long for the fluid to flow through Landon's short gut and into his diaper. Kathy changed the diaper. Then another. And another. Several times during the night, half-awake, I heard Kathy mumble, "I'm sorry, I'm sorry," while she wiped Landon's red bottom, and he cried in pain. She changed ten diapers that night.

At 4:30 a.m. I woke to the sound of gagging. Kathy held Landon while he vomited into a towel. "Too much formula," Kathy said. "Shelly warned me. It happens most nights."

I feared Landon would vomit again and aspirate – suck fluids into his lungs—so I stopped the formula pump and unhooked the tube from the G-tube. Then I grabbed a fresh towel and wiped vomit from his mattress before Kathy put him back in his crib.

After a year of watching Jeremiah and Shelly do it, Kathy and I had no problem managing the G-tube in Landon's stomach, but we still didn't feel skilled enough to handle the central line that pumped TPN into one of Landon's veins. At 6:00 a.m., while Kathy changed another diaper, I woke Jeremiah. He stopped the TPN, disconnected the lines, placed ethanol in the central line, capped the line, then stumbled back to bed. Kathy took Landon, ready to play again, to our living room. I crawled back in my bed for another hour of sleep. Jeremiah and Shelly slept until afternoon.

How did my son and daughter-in-law endure this every night? How much longer could they?

June 24, 2010, Jeremiah and Shelly drove Landon to Duke for the scheduled liver biopsy. Afterward, they met with the transplant team. Then Jeremiah called my cell. His voiced cracked, "They want to put Landon on the transplant list now."

I gasped. Was it time?

Chapter 22

Is it Time?

During the summer of 2010, I sweated over the decision we faced—put my grandson on the transplant list now, or wait?

If we placed Landon on the list and the transplant happened soon, he might be too small or weak to survive. But if we waited, any one of many things could kill him before he got bigger or stronger. The transplant team wanted to wait for the results of the liver biopsy before deciding if they should list Landon for a small intestine or the more daunting small intestine and liver. Their delay gave us several weeks to decide and prepare.

With the temperature at our mountain home ten to fifteen degrees cooler than at our son's home in Taylorsville, he and his family often stayed with us. The time together allowed us to discuss the recommendation from Duke. My son and daughter-in-law looked to me for advice.

In the fourteen months since Landon's birth, I had read everything I could find about pediatric intestinal transplants. I considered myself well educated on the subject. Still, my mind seesawed with conflicting thoughts and emotions.

Many nights, I tossed, turned, and sweated until the sheets were damp. On those nights, I prayed, "God, help us make the right decision. Give us a sign." I didn't expect God's hand to appear and write on a wall, or anything, but it might have helped.

After Landon's birth, I watched God intervene and no longer doubted His existence or His interest in our lives. I prayed for Him to heal Landon when he was sick and thanked God when Landon got better. Now, I cried out for guidance.

One evening, Jeremiah, Shelly, and Landon slept in our second bedroom. Roger and Ezekiel slept on the fold-out sofa sleeper in our living room.

While Kathy and I sat in bed, my wife thumbed the pages of a *Weight Watchers Magazine*, and I chuckled at the monologue of a late-night talk show host. A light breeze blew through the window and cooled our room.

Kathy laid the magazine on the bed. "We need more room."

"You want a king-size bed," I said, smiling.

"No, silly." She tapped my arm and grinned. "Space. Jeremiah and Shelly need help with Landon. When it comes time for the transplant, Roger and Ezekiel should live with us while Landon's in the hospital, and we still haven't decided what to do with your mother."

I didn't like where this conversation was going—my workshop. I frowned.

When I restored our old farmhouse, ten years earlier, I tore out one of the three bedrooms to make the living room bigger. At the same time, I constructed an eight-hundred-square-foot building beside the house to use as a workshop. In the far right corner of the building, I built a bathroom with a shower. I used about a quarter of the remaining space for my pursuits. I tied flies, and I made archery arrows for hunting. In the near left corner, a desk held ham radio equipment and also served as my office. The rest of the space we used for storage.

Kathy wanted me to pack my hobby supplies, get rid of the stored items, build bedrooms, and turn my workshop into a small house, a place for Jeremiah's family to stay. Reluctant, I slept on the idea.

The next morning at breakfast, I sketched on a napkin my idea for two bedrooms, a living room, and a galley kitchen. I showed it to Jeremiah. He stood beside the table and smiled.

"I can help." He placed his hands on his lower back. "My back still hurts, but if you want to do this, I'll help you build it."

I stood. "I do." I handed my empty plate to Kathy, who placed it in the dishwasher, then kissed me.

That afternoon I went to the local building supply store and purchased the materials we needed.

A week later, with the walls framed and the wiring in place, Jeremiah and I slid a sheet of drywall in place then took a break.

"Let's sit and drink water," I said.

My son sat on a five-gallon bucket of drywall putty and sipped from a plastic bottle. He leaned forward, placed his elbows on his knees, and lowered his head.

"Thinking about the transplant?" I said.

"It's all I have on my mind." He looked at the floor and shook his head. "Shelly thinks we should put Landon on the transplant list now."

"I understand why Duke wants to change the goal, but I'm not convinced," I said. "Maybe we should wait a little longer." I leaned against the wall and gulped water.

Jeremiah said, "If we do put him on the list, it could still take a long time to get a transplant. The average wait time is almost a year."

"But it could happen at any time." I looked at the construction in progress. "And, we're not ready."

With one hand on his lower back, Jeremiah eased off the bucket and stood. "Well, let's get ready. Let's get this done. I'll need to relax for a few days when we finish."

While Jeremiah and I worked on the new house, Shelly pursued an opportunity. She needed a job.

Because of Landon's frequent illnesses, it was difficult for Shelly to work, and she lost a couple of jobs. She needed a boss that understood and found that with Michael and Katy.

They had finished restorations on the old bowling alley

in Sparta, built an adjoining restaurant, and were looking for waitstaff. Shelly's experience and attitude got her the job. It didn't take long for the restaurant to become the most popular eating establishment in Sparta and the bowling alley a regular hangout for locals. Many of the customers knew about Landon and recognized Shelly. Those customers left generous tips. I'm not sure if they did it because of Landon or if they appreciated Shelly's excellent service. I think it was both.

After Jeremiah and I finished building the bedrooms, I purchased a couple of beds and found a used sofa sleeper for the living room. Jeremiah, Shelly, and the boys moved in.

We knew we could lose Landon at a young age. That knowledge gave us a desire to capture and preserve moments of his life. We took lots of pictures.

We were thrilled when a professional photographer from Matthews, North Carolina, Whitney, donated her services and did a photoshoot for Landon. She captured some beautiful pictures. They looked great on Landon's website, and we used them to design eye-catching flyers and brochures for the fundraisers. One adorns the cover of this book.

God brought Whitney into Landon's life to take the pictures we needed. Later, through Whitney, He would provide something even more valuable.

After the photoshoot, Jeremiah, Shelly, and Landon went home to Taylorsville, where the home nurse, made a scheduled visit. She drew blood, recorded Landon's vital signs, and weighed him.

Jeremiah called with good news. "Landon has gained five pounds in the past month. He weighs twenty-two pounds. He's never gained that much in one month."

I raised my hands and said, "Thank you."

It wasn't writing on the wall, but Landon had passed a significant threshold, twenty pounds, needed to get him on the transplant list.

Kathy and I discussed having a party, but our celebratory mood didn't last long. That evening, Landon developed a low-grade temperature. The previous week, the pediatrician had given him another round of infant vaccinations. The doctor warned Shelly the shots might cause a slight fever. Not sure if the shots caused it or if something else did, Jeremiah and Shelly watched their son through the night. The next morning, with his temperature near 102, they rushed to Duke.

In Landon's hospital room, again, the familiar routine unfolded, a nurse inserted an IV, administered antibiotics, and drew blood for lab cultures.

The lab soon determined that the same bacteria, which caused the infection in March and again in late April, also caused this one. We thought the ethanol had killed the "nasty bug" - as the surgeon first described it. It didn't. The bacteria must have hidden in Landon's central line and re-emerged. It seemed my fears were coming true. If he couldn't beat the infection again, he was going to lose this line. With only two access sites remaining, I shuddered at the thought of using one of those.

In the hospital, Jeremiah and Shelly tended to Landon. They kept him cool, managed the G-tube feedings, changed diapers, and entertained their irritable son. When exhausted, they took turns and slept in a recliner in the hospital room.

Four days later, Landon's fever remained, and one of our fears came true.

The transplant surgeon and the nurse who two months earlier had shown Jeremiah and Shelly how to use ethanol in the line, entered Landon's room. "I'm afraid the bacteria have grown stronger, more resistant. We must remove the central line now," the surgeon motioned toward the nurse. "She will take it out."

Ten minutes later, Jeremiah called our shop.

Kathy answered. She closed her eyes and shook her head.

The look on her face told me all I needed to know. I hung my head and swallowed hard.

Three days later, Kathy and I drove Roger and Ezekiel to Durham for a visit. We arrived late in the evening, near the end of visiting hours.

Landon's temperature was still high, but lower than when his parents rushed him to the hospital. Our grandson smiled when we entered the room. He tried to stand in his bed, but an IV in his foot kept him from doing so. Roger and Ezekiel sat on each side of the bed. Roger played a tune on Landon's toy guitar. Ezekiel held an orange stuffed Tigger tiger and bounced it on the mattress. Landon smiled. The brothers played until time for us to leave.

Kathy decided to spend the night at the hospital with Shelly and Landon. Jeremiah, the older boys, and I walked to a hotel and got a room. Fully clothed, Jeremiah plopped on a bed and went to sleep in minutes. Roger and Ezekiel went to the hotel pool and swam for an hour before bedtime.

The next morning, Shelly and I switched places.

When Landon's doctor arrived for morning rounds, we discovered that our grandson's temperature was normal. Kathy begged permission from the doctor to take Landon on a tour of the hospital. She agreed. Kathy dressed our grandson, and then I strapped him into his stroller. To protect the IV in Landon's foot, Kathy knelt and wrapped a disposable diaper around it. It looked like a white boot.

Landon gazed at his grandmother and said, "Mawmaw."

I'm not sure if a beam of light through the window caused my wife's face to glow or if our grandson's voice did. Kathy knelt and handed Landon his "passy." Ready for the adventure, he popped it in his mouth and clapped his hands.

Kathy pushed the stroller, and I trailed close, with the IV stand on wheels. In the halls, I nodded, acknowledged the sympathetic looks, and smiled. Kathy smiled. Moon-eyed, Landon strained against the stroller belt. On the fourth floor, we discovered an aquarium; on the roof, a helicopter; and in the main lobby, a water fountain.

Landon leaned forward and looked at the bubbling water. A girl about five years old walked to the edge of the fountain and tossed a coin in. I placed a penny in my grandson's hand and made a throwing action. He flung the coin, smiled, and extended his hand for another. I gave him one. He threw it. I closed my eyes, made a wish—a prayer—and with a backhand motion, like you would throw a frisbee, I let go of a coin. It skipped across the water, then floated to the bottom and landed on top of a thousand other wishes.

The next day a surgeon placed a new central line in a vein in Landon's neck. To keep the site sanitary and away from my grandson's hands, the doctor tunneled the line under the skin on the left side of Landon's chest. A t-shirt covered the exit site and helped to protect it. This more invasive procedure caused several days of pain for Landon. He cried often.

With one available access site remaining, I prayed, "God, let this site last until my grandson gets a transplant."

The time had come to place Landon on the transplant list. I knew it. Still, we weren't ready. We didn't have everything in place, and we hadn't raised enough money.

About this time, a group of volunteers approached me with an idea for another COTA fundraiser, a Bowl-A-Rama.

Chapter 23

The Bowl-a-Rama and the Seizure

"What the heck is a Bowl-A-Rama?" I said.

A pink-faced lady grinned and said, "It's a day of fundraising centered around bowling." Her eyes twinkled.

I should have figured it had something to do with bowling by the shirts that she and her husband wore—yellow button-downs with brown collars and a graphic of a bowling ball knocking down pins on the left breasts.

I loved the idea: a fundraiser involving the bowling community. Michael and Katy, Shelly's employers, had already agreed to donate the use of the bowling alley.

"Go for it," I said and smiled.

Soon, the energy, excitement, and joy of this couple spread to Landon's other COTA volunteers.

A week later, a group met at our shop and planned a youth and adult tournament, a raffle, and an auction. In the weeks that followed, they recruited bowlers and bowling teams from the local leagues, from Sparta and surrounding towns as well. A group of ladies from the wellness center took the lead in selling raffle tickets for a two-night family vacation at an rustic indoor waterpark resort near Charlotte, North Carolina.

We collected donated auction items and displayed them at our fabric showroom.

Our hometown newspaper, *The Alleghany News*, published an article about the fundraiser, and I posted regular updates on Landon's blog.

Like previous fundraisers, the people and circumstances needed for a successful event seemed to fall in place.

The entry requirement for youth to enter the tournament was for the child to bring in donations they had collected—any amount. A couple of dozen kids signed up.

Teams of adults could enter by donating $100. Teams, with names like "Hammack's Hammers" (a construction crew), and "The BCB Bombers" (truck drivers), signed up. With each raffle ticket sold, each item donated for the auction, and each team registered for the tournament, the anticipation and excitement of the event, a week away, grew. I prayed the Bowl-A-Rama would raise a lot of money for my grandson.

Landon remained in the hospital in Durham and continued to recover from the latest line placement. The doctors discharged him two days before the fundraiser. We hoped he would feel well enough to attend.

Saturday morning, July 24, the day of the Bowl-A-Rama, one of the ladies who helped organize the youth tournament stood in front of the bowling lanes and looked at her watch. Six children stood in front of their lanes, bowling balls in hand. Other children scrambled to choose bowling balls from the racks.

Seconds before 11:00 a.m., the lady held her hand in the air and said, "Five, four, three, two, one, go," and dropped her hand to start the Bowl-A-Rama.

Each child bowled a game and received a piece of pizza, popcorn, and a drink.

At 1:00 p.m., the children cleared out, and the first ball from an adult bowler roared down a lane and slammed into the pins with a force that jarred my teeth.

A few minutes after the adult tournament got underway, Shelly arrived with Landon. Still recovering from the painful surgery, he rested on his mother's hip and laid his head on her shoulder. Shelly stood with Kathy and me behind a row of spectator seats and a short wall that separated the bowling lanes from the arcade area and provided a view of the lanes. A few bowlers realized that Landon had arrived and waved at him. Shelly held Landon's arm and helped him wave back. He looked confused, and the sound of balls smashing into pins startled him.

The event organizers and some of the bowlers who weren't yet bowling came over to greet Landon. I snapped pictures. Shelly was friendly, as always, but I detected a nervousness in her laugh, and she pulled away when a man attempted to touch Landon. She feared her son might pick up another bug, so thirty minutes after they arrived, she took Landon home.

At 7:00 p.m., an auctioneer banged a gavel to start the auction. Pretty soon, the call of one of the three auctioneers filled the building. We were overwhelmed by the number of items donated—tools, prints, glassware, furniture, canned goods, baked goods, and more.

I held the merchandise in the air for display and shouted "Yes" as loud as I could when I saw someone make a bid with a card, a finger, or a wink.

When the bidding on a bowl donated by a local potter stopped short of the actual value, the auctioneer stopped his chant and said, "Remember folks, this is for Landon."

The bidding resumed, and the bowl sold for twice its value. The little gray-haired lady who won the bid stood and hugged my neck when I handed her the mixing bowl. I swallowed hard and choked back tears.

Two hours into the auction, one of the auctioneers interrupted the sale and asked a girl in the audience to draw a ticket from the box of raffle tickets. A woman in the crowd jumped and clapped when she won the trip to the water park. Later, when she and her family redeemed the vacation, the resort upgraded the rooms because the package raised money for a COTA patient.

Like the previous fundraisers, I felt God's love for my grandson through every person who participated. The money raised at the Bowl-A-Rama pushed the total donated to more than $24,000.

A week after the event, we were still bubbling with excitement when the seizure happened.

Kathy says Landon acted like he didn't feel well that morning, but it didn't alarm her. He played in our living room and followed her around the kitchen and dining room while she cleaned and cooked. He pulled cans out of a cabinet and stacked them on the floor until Kathy hauled him back to the sofa for another diaper change.

Jeremiah and Shelly, who had slept late that morning, walked through the front door while Kathy was changing the diaper. Landon smiled at his parents. If his bottom hurt when Kathy wiped him, he didn't react. When Kathy finished, she held her grandson in her arms and placed her face close to his.

Landon made a low gurgling noise, almost a hiss. His body stiffened then shook.

Kathy looked at his face and gasped when his eyes rolled back. She placed him on her lap and screamed, "Landon."

Shelly knelt beside her convulsing son and cradled his head in her hands.

Kathy remembers the seizure lasting for several minutes; Jeremiah and Shelly say no more than thirty seconds. When it ended, Landon whimpered then cried. Shelly took her son from Kathy's lap, looked into his eyes, then held him to her chest, and rocked him from side to side.

Kathy lowered her face into her cupped hands and cried.

Jeremiah used our home phone and called 911. He then called me at our business in town, three miles away.

The ambulance arrived a few minutes before me. I jumped from my truck and ran toward the emergency vehicle and the flashing red lights. A female EMT carried Landon to the ambulance and strapped him on a gurney. Kathy followed, wiping tears.

I grabbed her. "What happened?"

She sobbed and said, "I thought he was dying in my arms."

The ambulance driver and I helped Kathy climb into the back of the vehicle. She sat beside Landon and held his hand.

Jeremiah shouted to me as he climbed into his car, "His fever is almost 104. We've got to go before he has another seizure."

He and Shelly followed the ambulance out of our driveway.

Roger and Ezekiel, who were playing video games next door when the seizure happened, stood in the yard and watched the vehicles leave. I told them to get into my truck.

A few minutes later, I arrived at the hospital in Sparta with the older brothers in tow.

Jeremiah, red-cheeked and watery-eyed, met us in the parking lot outside of the emergency room. He gulped hard. "They've called for a helicopter from Duke."

I placed my hand on my forehead, "Do the doctors think he is so sick that they need to fly him out of here?"

"They must," Jeremiah said. "The doctor said something about septic shock, and the chopper could be here in less than an hour." My son turned and looked at the helicopter landing pad in a field beside the hospital and then shook his head. In the distance, thunder rumbled.

A few minutes later, Duke called back and told us the helicopter couldn't come. A line of severe thunderstorms over the Tennessee border was moving east toward us and made it unsafe for the helicopter to fly to Sparta. Duke dispatched an ambulance instead. It would arrive in about two hours.

While we waited for the ambulance, the doctors in Sparta worked to control the fever and hoped to prevent another seizure. Landon's temperature had risen fast several times before, but this fever was different, and we were scared. Shelly and Kathy stayed in the emergency room and comforted Landon. Roger and Ezekiel watched television in the waiting room. Jeremiah and I went to our house, packed a couple of bags of clothing and toiletries, then returned to the hospital in our car. He and I paced in the parking lot and speculated about what caused the seizure.

"I thought God was protecting Landon," Jeremiah said and shook his head.

I stopped walking and looked at my son. "Maybe He is. Landon will soon be on his way to one of the best hospitals in the world."

Jeremiah removed his ball cap, rubbed the top of his nearly bald head, and looked at the sky. "Then why did God let this happen in the first place?"

Lightning struck a mountain top close to the hospital, and we ran for the emergency room door.

We stood behind the glass door and watched the thunderstorm roar across the mountains and into town. I took a deep breath and wondered if the storm would slow the ambulance. It didn't. Thirty minutes later, the emergency vehicle arrived.

The storm continued with waves of windblown rain. Sheltered by a roof at the emergency room doors, the paramedics loaded Landon into the ambulance. With two medics on board, they didn't have room for a parent. The vehicle pulled away from the hospital—Jeremiah and Shelly, with Roger and Ezekiel, close behind. Kathy and I followed both.

"Go," I said three times and pounded on the steering wheel. "Why don't they turn on the lights and siren and go faster?"

"Calm down," Kathy said. "They've got things under control."

During the drive down the mountain, the rain fell harder, and the fog rolled in. Kathy insisted that I drive slower. I did and soon lost sight of Jeremiah's vehicle and the ambulance. When we arrived in Durham, a little before dark, the rain had stopped, and Landon was already in a room.

The doctor suspected another infection, nine days after my grandson beat the last one. With a new IV and antibiotics flowing, Landon didn't feel much like playing, but he recognized where he was and seemed right at home. He unpacked his stuffed animals and settled back to watch cartoons, surrounded by his soft furry friends.

Although the medicines the doctor in Sparta gave Landon helped to reduce his fever, the nurse at Duke still got a reading of 102.

I figured that the same old bacteria that caused the last infections also caused this one. It didn't. When a doctor told us what the lab found, my knees wobbled. Klebsiella, a healthcare-associated, antibiotic-resistant killer, sometimes referred to as a superbug.

As the term "healthcare-associated" implies, klebsiella infects patients who are in a healthcare facility, such as a rest home or a hospital. More than likely, this bug infected Landon during his last admission.

I had read about this bacterium on the blogs of other short-bowel children and how it contributed to the deaths of several. The name—klebsiella—sounds like the name of an evil witch.

The bacteria revealed its power in how fast it caused Landon's temperature to spike. Fast enough to cause a seizure. From the pictures of Klebsiella, I saw on the Internet, I imagined this elongated purple microscopic creature with fangs lurking under the hospital bed waiting to attack my grandson.

When I described Klebsiella to Shelly and told her how Landon might have acquired it, the momma bear in her emerged. She removed a small plastic canister of antiseptic wipes that she carried in Landon's diaper bag and proceeded to sanitize the room. My daughter-in-law wiped the doorknobs, the sink, the bed rails, and every exposed surface. She wouldn't let anyone in the room unless they first used an antiseptic gel on their hands. She scolded nurses and doctors if they forgot.

To fight the resistant bacteria, the doctor prescribed a combination of powerful antibiotics.

Kathy and I couldn't afford a hotel room for more than one night, so the next day, we returned home and took Roger and Ezekiel with us.

The medicine worked. A couple of days later, Landon's fever returned to near normal. He sat in his bed, played with his toys, and watched a DVD of his favorite cartoon character—Olivia.

Four days into this admission, Jeremiah and Shelly met with the transplant team and officially gave the okay to place Landon on the transplant list. Even though he didn't lose this central line and he still had one more site on the other side of his neck, we couldn't risk waiting any longer.

The tests the doctors did the previous month confirmed the TPN had damaged Landon's liver but not enough to require a liver transplant. The transplant team decided to list Landon for a small intestine, and not a multi-visceral small intestine and liver transplant. In a couple more weeks, after the transplant team submitted the paperwork, the United Network for Organ Sharing (UNOS) would place Landon on the waiting list.

Five days later, the transplant surgeon determined the Klebsiella infection was gone. Jeremiah and Shelly could bring Landon home.

When they arrived back on the mountain, they found another person living there—my mother.

Chapter 24

The Caregiver and the Transplant List

When my mother came to live with us, Kathy became Mom's primary caregiver.

Mom brought changes to our lives. Kathy and I no longer worked together at our shop, and my wife didn't leave the house without someone to watch my mother. I liked having my mom with us, but it added a layer of stress to our already stressful lives.

To make room for my mother, we removed the furniture from the largest of our two bedrooms and ordered a hospital bed, wheelchair, and a lift. Before our order arrived, Kathy rolled up her sleeves, mopped, cleaned, and sanitized the empty room. While I emptied a bucket of dirty mop water, I thought of how God blessed me with a hard-working, compassionate wife and smiled. When a local home healthcare agency delivered the items, Kathy watched while they assembled them, and listened when they explained how to use everything.

I think my wife enjoyed taking care of my mother. She rose early each morning and hummed along to music on the radio in Mother's room while she tended to Mom. Kathy carried on cheerful conversations, even when my mother didn't always reply. Mom didn't talk much anymore. But, I think she liked living at our home. Over time, the muscles in her face and jaws became rigid, but she sometimes forced a smile, especially when Landon came to visit.

After our grandson returned home from his last admission at Duke, Kathy often tended to both him and Mom, cleaned the house, and cooked meals, all at the same time. I marveled at how she accomplished her work with a cheerful attitude. And, her responsibilities weren't limited to the home. We still had a business to run, and I couldn't do it without help from Kathy.

When we had complicated sewing work to do, I could sew, but not with the same skill as my wife, I would go home and sit with my mother while Kathy went to our shop and worked.

Late in the afternoon of August 25, I worked in our kitchen preparing hamburger patties for the grill while Kathy tended to Mom in the bedroom. Jeremiah and Shelly, with Landon in her arms, rushed through the front door and to the kitchen. The commotion alerted Kathy, and she followed the sound of excited voices.

"Duke finished the paperwork," Jeremiah said. "Landon is officially on the transplant list."

Kathy's face flushed red, and eyes teared. She smiled, then covered her mouth with a hand.

A fullness in my chest moved to my throat. I swallowed hard. Landon could get a transplant soon, yet thoughts of the complicated, risky surgery overwhelmed my wife and me.

"Now what do we do?" I said, wiping my eyes with the back of my greasy hands.

"We need to have bags packed, ready to go," Jeremiah said. "The call could come at any time. When it does, we need to get Landon to Duke within four hours."

Kathy took Landon from Shelly's arms and squeezed him.

I returned to my hamburger patties and the grill where I imagined a call from Duke and a mad dash to the hospital. The lump in my throat turned to butterflies in my stomach.

Later that evening, in bed, I prayed, "God, please make an organ available for Landon." The prayer bothered me. Had I prayed for another child's death so Landon could receive a small intestine? I didn't intend to, but in my mind, that's how the prayer sounded.

I tried another approach. "God, if a child dies who matches Landon, I pray that You will guide the parents in a decision to donate the child's organs, and my grandson will receive a perfect small intestine." I prayed the same prayer each night while we waited for a call from Duke.

Three days after Duke placed Landon on the transplant list, he woke with another fever. He didn't have another seizure, but his parents rushed him back to Duke anyway.

The wicked witch—Klebsiella—had returned. Landon wanted her to go away. Unlike other times, Landon became angry when a nurse took him to a room. He cried and slapped at the nurse when she attempted to insert an IV. When Shelly tried to comfort him, he mustered all the strength a sixteen-month-old could hit his mother, and then wailed when she restrained him.

Landon battled with Shelly and two nurses until they completed the routine to prepare him for another fight against the bacteria. Still not happy, he curled in the bed, closed his tear-filled eyes, and went to sleep.

Landon awoke in a better mood. He gathered his stuffed animals around him and let the antibiotics fight the battle.

This infection didn't get as bad as the previous one or as scary. Three days after being admitted, Landon's temperature returned to normal. Four days later, the doctor discharged him, and his parents drove him home.

We rushed to their recently purchased minivan when they returned. While Kathy and Shelly carried Landon, his diaper bag, and the pump bag to the house, I stood at the back of the vehicle. Jeremiah walked around the side.

"I hope Klebsiella is gone for good," I said.

Jeremiah opened the rear hatch, then raised his arms and stretched. "Me too. We are tired."

I reached in the vehicle and removed a suitcase. "You and Shelly get some rest. We'll watch Landon this evening. Besides, we missed him while he was gone and would enjoy taking care of him."

We sent them off to rest, and Kathy and I played with our grandson until bedtime.

The next day, my wife and I knelt in front of a flower bed. We shared some playful banter as we weeded, giving us a moment of joy.

Kathy scooped a handful of dirt, threw it at me, and smiled just as I reached for the water hose, grinned, and pointed the nozzle her way.

The door to the small house opened.

Jeremiah rushed out with a suitcase in his hand. "They've got a transplant," he shouted. "We've got to go now." He ran to the van, opened the rear hatch, and threw the suitcase in.

I dropped the water hose and jumped to my feet. "We aren't ready," I said. "We don't have our bags packed, and we don't have anyone to take care of Mom." My heart thumped while I helped Kathy stand.

Shelly walked out of the house with Landon on her hip and tears dripping from her cheeks. She carried Landon's black TPN pump bag in her hand, and his diaper bag hung from her shoulder. I ran to her and took the diaper bag. Kathy grabbed Landon and held him close.

Jeremiah's phone rang. He answered right away. "That's okay. … We understand." After disconnecting, he exhaled long and slow and looked at us. "The transplant doctor rejected the organ. She said it didn't match close enough."

Kathy held Landon and cried.

Jeremiah and Shelly, with heads lowered, unloaded the van.

I sat on the steps to the house, diaper bag in hand, and looked at the ground. My heartbeat slowed. "Maybe the next one will be a perfect match, and we'll be ready."

It wasn't. And we weren't.

Two weeks later, Jeremiah and I drove to a Lowe's in the neighboring town of West Jefferson, about an hour away. I purchased plumbing materials for the small house. Before heading home, we stopped at a KFC for lunch. We sat at a table and took a few bites of chicken.

Jeremiah's phone rang. His eyes widened in a look of shock. Then he nodded and grinned. "We'll get there as quick as we can." He looked at me. "They've got a matching organ. We've got to go."

We threw our meal in the trash, ran to my truck, and sped out of the parking lot.

Jeremiah called Shelly. "Get Landon ready. If we hit any traffic, we'll not get to Durham within four hours." He pulled the phone away from his ear, looked at the screen. "Shelly, Duke is calling. Hold on." He tapped, listened, then said, "That's okay. We understand." My son looked at the floorboard.

I eased my foot from the accelerator. The truck slowed to the speed limit.

The transplant doctor rejected the organ again.

"Do you want to stop and get something else for lunch?" I said.

"No, I don't feel like eating." He closed his eyes and leaned his head back on the headrest.

After that day, because we feared not getting Landon to Duke soon enough when the next call came, we didn't travel far from the house.

At home, Landon kept his grandmother busy, and his great grandmother entertained. He often played on Mom's bed.

On September 24, Jeremiah disconnected the TPN from the central line. He noticed difficulty when he used a syringe to withdraw fluids. He examined the line and then pushed the plunger to force fluids back into it. A bulge appeared in the plastic tubing about four inches away from where the line entered Landon's chest. Landon must have kinked and damaged it during play. With just one other access site remaining, we didn't want to lose this one. Jeremiah secured the line with tape and a popsicle stick. Then he and Shelly loaded Landon in the van for another trip to Duke and a mission to save Landon's central line.

The commotion around Landon and his sudden departure alarmed my mother.

In a feeble voice, she asked, "Is it time for his transplant?" She still understood, at least at times, that Landon needed a transplant.

"No, he needs to go to the hospital, but he'll be okay," I said with uncertainty.

We prayed Landon wouldn't lose this line like the one he

lost nine months earlier under similar circumstances. He didn't. The repair worked. That evening, Landon returned home, having overcome yet another threat.

Broken central lines and microscopic organisms weren't the only threats to Landon and his family that fall. Not all men have hearts filled with love and a desire to help other people. Evil exists, and my son and daughter-in-law came face to face with it.

Three weeks after the line repair, Jeremiah and Shelly drove Landon to Durham for a scheduled visit. After the appointment, they drove to their home in Taylorsville to retrieve a few items they wanted to take to their new home in the mountains.

They pulled into the driveway of their secluded home. A pickup truck sat in front of the house with some of their belongings in the back. The house door stood open.

Jeremiah and Shelly slipped out of their vehicle, leaving Landon asleep in his car seat. My son didn't see anyone around. He approached the truck, reached through the driver's open window, and removed the keys. He and Shelly entered the front door and heard voices of men at the rear of the house. Shelly dialed 911. Jeremiah grabbed two knives from the kitchen cabinet and surprised three men. With a knife in each hand, my son held the robbers at bay. The deputy who patrolled the neighborhood raced to Jeremiah's house and arrived in less than five minutes. Others followed. The deputies handcuffed the men and took them to jail. A few years later, a homeowner shot and killed one of the three men during another attempted burglary.

Still shaking when they arrived at our home, Jeremiah and

Shelly told us what happened. We talked about all the what-ifs and how the situation could have turned out much worse.

"Thank God it didn't," I said. "An angel must have been watching over you."

Kathy lowered her head and moped back to Mom's room.

I followed. "What's wrong? They're okay."

"I know, I'm just tired, but your mom has bedsores."

I looked at Mom, sleeping in her bed.

The next day Mom's doctor visited - something that still occurred in the mountains in the early 2000s. After he examined her, he asked Kathy and me to step outside, where Mom couldn't hear us.

He looked at Kathy. "How are you doing?"

"I'm fine," she said and averted her eyes.

She wasn't, and the doctor could tell. The stress of taking care of Mom and worrying about our family was catching up with my wife.

"I'm going to call hospice and request that they send some nurses to help you," the doctor said.

Three days later, an administrator from hospice and two nurses showed up at our house. After they evaluated Mom, they worked out a schedule to come to our home three days each week and help Kathy.

During the visits, the nurses monitored Mom's vital signs and diabetes. They also showed Kathy easier and better ways to care for my mother. The interaction with the nurses cheered Kathy. Soon Mom's bedsore healed, and my wife's energy returned. She hurried around the house and hummed while she pampered my mother and cooked for the holidays

That Thanksgiving, unlike the previous year, when Landon was in the hospital, and we had to delay our meal, our loved ones arrived on time for the feast.

Before we ate, the family asked me to pray. We all bowed our heads, and I gave thanks for our time together. Before I asked for a blessing on the food, I thanked God for watching over Landon. That's when I realized the day marked three months since the doctors placed our grandson on the transplant list, and still, we hadn't found a transplant. Kathy wrapped her arm around my back and laid her head on my shoulder while I struggled to finish the prayer. When I did, Shelly handed out napkins, and we wiped our tears.

Kathy sniffled and said, "God has taken care of Landon, and He will continue to do so. Now, let's eat."

The next day, Black Friday, my wife, along with Shelly and Jessica, hit the stores in search of Christmas bargains. I stayed at home with Mom. With Kathy taking care of Mom and only working a few hours each week, we didn't have a lot of money to spend and again couldn't afford to give our grandchildren much for Christmas. We hoped Santa would show up. And he did in a big way.

In early December, Shelly answered a call from the pharmacy

in Winston-Salem that had provided Landon's TPN and medical supplies since his birth. The caller told Shelly that each Christmas, the employees at the pharmacy selected a patient and provided Christmas gifts for the patient and the patient's family. This year they chose Landon and his family.

The caller instructed Shelly to prepare a wish list for Landon, each of his brothers, and his parents, and to include one special gift for each.

Three days before Christmas, a man backed a green pickup truck with a camper shell on the bed to the front door of our shop in Sparta. A burly man with gray hair and a full white beard stepped out of the truck. He wore a red sweatshirt and a black cowboy hat.

He didn't say, "Ho, ho, ho," but the man from the pharmacy extended his hand and opened the back of the truck.

"Wow," I said, stepping back. Not wanting to cry in front of the big man, I choked back tears.

Wrapped packages filled the truck.

I helped unload the gifts, shook the man's hand again, and thanked him before he left. I don't remember hugging the man, but I should have. I stored the packages at the shop because the tree wasn't ready at the small house.

Shelly waited to decorate a Christmas tree until two days before Christmas, when Roger, who now lived with Shelly's brother so he could continue to attend high school in Taylorsville, arrived home for the holidays.

Christmas Eve, with the decorations in place at both the small house and our home, Kathy and I prepared another feast. We baked pies and cookies. Kathy made banana pudding. My favorite. In the evening, I purchased a ham at the grocery store and then went to the shop where I helped Jeremiah load the gifts from the pharmacy into his van. That evening, after the boys went to bed, their parents slipped the packages under the tree. Kathy tucked Mom into bed. Then my wife and I sat close to our warm wood stove, listened to the fire crackle, and watched Christmas movies.

Christmas morning, Landon's second, Kathy and I entered the small house. Landon shouted, "Bike, bike, bike," and showed us his new tricycle. The older boys talked in excited tones while they unwrapped their gifts. Roger got a new cell phone. Ezekiel received an iPod. The family, an X-box electronic game. Jeremiah and Shelly, together on the sofa, smiled while they watched their sons unwrap gifts. My treat came in the afternoon when our family gathered for another big meal.

We gorged, and later ate leftovers for most of the next week. I must have gained ten pounds in one week.

We received our Christmas wishes, all but one, a transplant for Landon. Still, the year ended with us fat and happy to have our family close.

Chapter 25

Running and Praying

After a gluttonous holiday season, Kathy and I decided to make losing weight a resolution for the new year. To set the goal was one thing, to achieve it another.

I didn't have a plan until Kathy convinced me to join her at a Weight Watchers meeting. There, I met Sherry, the local leader, who explained the program.

I love a challenge, and losing weight became one. So, after the meeting, Kathy and I took inventory of the items in our pantry and threw out everything with too many points—Weight Watchers count points, not calories. We trashed the sugary cereals, potato chips, and soft drinks, then went to the grocery store and purchased foods we could use to prepare healthy meals. I cut out my sweet snacks and restricted my portion sizes at meals. My stomach protested until I learned that most fruits and vegetables were zero points, so I grazed on those. The growling in my belly soon stopped.

A week later, we returned to a meeting. I had lost two pounds. I stepped off the scale and looked at the floor. I'm not sure how much I expected to lose, but two pounds didn't sound like much.

Sherry must have seen the disappointment on my face. "If you exercise, you'll lose more," she said.

Several evenings the next week, when it wasn't too cold, didn't rain, or snow, and Jeremiah or Jessica could stay with Mom, Kathy and I went to the track at the local high school and walked.

Behind the goal post at the far end of the track, I gasped for air. "Slow down. Are you trying to kill me?"

"Maybe," Kathy said. "But you should walk fast if you want to burn calories."

"Huh? I thought we weren't counting calories."

"You know what I mean," my wife said and walked faster.

Her short legs outpaced mine two to one. She exaggerated the swing of her arms, and I struggled to keep up.

"Why don't we just run?" I said, and puffed.

She looked at me and grinned. "I'd bet you couldn't run a half a lap." My wife knew how to push my buttons—always had.

So, I did, I ran one-half of a lap—one-eighth of a mile. Panting and shaking, I stopped. My legs wobbled. I held my hand to my stinging throat and sucked cold air into my burning lungs. I walked until my heart rate slowed, and my lungs stopped hurting. Then I jogged until I caught Kathy. With my hands in the air, I shouted, "I did it," then bent over, placed my hands on my knees, and coughed until I gagged.

"Barely," my wife said and laughed.

That was all it took to get me started running, and she knew it.

Meeting Kathy at the track in the evenings became the highlight of my day. I came from our shop, and my wife came from home. The walks gave both of us a way to relieve some of the stress. A little each day, I increased the distance I ran. A few weeks later, in early February, I ran four laps—a mile—without stopping or vomiting. I celebrated by running to the top of the concrete bleachers then jumping with my fist in the air, like Rocky. Kathy stood on the track at the bottom of the bleachers and clapped.

Counting points and exercising became part of our everyday routine. The weight came off a little at a time. After six weeks on Weight Watchers, Kathy and I went to another meeting. My wife had lost almost twenty pounds, and I lost a little more. We high-fived and hugged. The women in the meeting clapped when Sherry announced our weight loss.

She then said, "Tell us about your exercise routine."

"Running on the track is okay," I said. "But going around and around gets a little boring. I want to get out on the roads, but I don't know good roads to run on."

Sherry smiled. "My husband, Chuck, is a runner. He knows where to run. I'll introduce you."

The next Saturday, I met Chuck—a man about my age, mid-fifties, but with the body of a runner and a smiling face that radiated a healthy glow—at the Little Glade Mill Pond on the Blue Ridge Parkway. We ran north on the scenic route for two miles, then turned around and headed back toward the millpond.

While we ran, I told Chuck about my grandson and how we continued to wait for a transplant. Chuck wiped a tear from the corner of his eye. When we arrived back at our vehicles, he asked if he could pray for Landon. We bowed our heads, and sweat dripped from my chin. Chuck prayed and wiped more tears.

Six months had passed since the doctors placed my grandson on the transplant list, but still, no transplant. And we hadn't received more false alarm calls, the repair to Landon's central line held, and he hadn't been sick.

Until Thursday morning, February 24, 2011. That morning, I sat at our dining room table and ate a bowl of oatmeal with sliced bananas and walnuts, all worth four points. I smiled when Shelly came in with Landon on her hip.

"What do you think of his first haircut?" she said, and ran her fingers through what remained of Landon's red curls.

I faked a smile but shook my head. Not that his hair was too short or looked terrible, but the shorter hair made his face look slender, sick.

I slid my chair back, stood, leaned in, and kissed Landon. He wrapped his arms around my neck and hugged, something he hadn't done before. His warm face pressed against my cheek. He released and rested his head on his mother's shoulder.

"Is he okay?" I said and looked at his pale face. Dark circles surrounded his blue eyes.

"I don't think he feels well," my daughter-in-law said and touched his cheek with the back of her hand. "He's warm."

Kathy came from Mom's room and helped Shelly take Landon's temperature. She looked at the thermometer, placed her hand on her cheek, and said, "Oh crap, 102."

An hour later, she kissed her sick grandson, then stood on the porch, wiped tears, and waved while Jeremiah and Shelly left our home to drive Landon to Duke.

Six months had passed since his last fever, and we feared another bacterial infection—possibly klebsiella. It wasn't. Twenty-four hours passed, and nothing grew in the lab cultures.

Three days later, I scratched my forehead when Jeremiah called and told us that our grandson's temperature remained elevated, and the doctors still didn't know what caused the fever. Why hadn't the antibiotics worked?

Landon grew restless and tossed his stuffed animals to the floor, then cried until his parents put them back in his bed. A few minutes later, he did it again. Shelly read to him until her son pushed the book away. He watched a video of *Toy Story* over and over.

A book fell from the bed. "Oh crap," Landon said, his grandmother's contribution to his vocabulary.

The next day the doctor discovered a reason for my grandson's fever—influenza type B. We should have figured, most of the population of Sparta was sick with the flu, including Landon's cousins and a brother. A day later, I became ill. The emergency room at the hospital in Sparta confirmed influenza. The home health nurse gave both Mom and Kathy a flu shot months earlier. They didn't get sick. Landon received a flu shot in the fall, yet he still got the flu. The doctor at Duke told Shelly the flu shot prevented her son from getting sicker.

Landon fought to overcome the flu, and with the help of IV fluids, he did. Kathy hugged and kissed him when he returned home. Still recovering from the virus, I kept my distance.

I soon felt better but missed more than a week of running while sick. Eager to run again, I called Chuck and asked him to meet me on the Parkway.

For me, the first three miles of a run hurt. I struggled. But after the warmup, the pain went away. I breathed deeper, my heart rate slowed, and I ran faster. During the run, Chuck and I talked about my new-found sport.

"I'm training to run the New River Marathon, a month from now." Chuck stared at the road ahead with a look of determination. "I plan to run fourteen miles in a couple of days, then a twenty-miler in a couple of weeks."

We chugged along and climbed a hill.

At the top, I said, "How do you run such long distances? How do you stay motivated?" I sipped from a water bottle, then wiped the sweat from my brow.

"I pray," Chuck said and smiled. "While I run, I talk to God." He pointed toward the sky, then ran off the road and into the bushes for a personal pit stop.

I continued to run. Chuck caught up with me a quarter of a mile later.

"There's a half-marathon at New River," Chuck said. "Why don't you sign up? I think you can do it."

I looked at my legs. "I don't know if I'm ready."

"Pray about it," Chuck said.

We separated and ran in the grass on the shoulder of the road while a car passed. I thought about what Chuck said—the half marathon and praying. We ran in silence until we finished the six miles. Before we left the parking lot at the millpond, Chuck prayed for Landon, again, and for me. A weird feeling came over me. I felt like something, or somebody, led me to this point in time and this place. I saw how events connected—the weight loss journey, running, meeting Chuck. I looked in his eyes, smiled, and nodded yes.

A few days later, I sat in a chair in our living room and laced my shoes for a run on a trail around our property. Kathy laid Landon on the sofa to change his diaper.

He looked different, drained, tired. The fight to survive almost two years without a small intestine had taken its toll. My grandson's rosy cheeks were now pale—ashen. His little, gaunt face framed dark circled eyes. I took a deep breath and exhaled.

Kathy removed the diaper, then wiped his bottom. He screamed the same ear-piercing scream we often heard. I grimaced and tried to block the sound. I wondered if Landon thought the painful diaper changes were a punishment. What I heard next, I couldn't ignore.

"I sorry, I sorry," Landon said while he squirmed and screamed.

They were the same words his mother and grandmother used to comfort him during the torturous diaper changes. Now they were his.

Tears blurred my eyes and streamed down my cheeks. I ran from the house, from the screams, and took up the trail. How much more could my grandson endure?

A light rain fell. The trail led through open meadows, and the wet grass soaked my shoes. I ran. In the forest, raindrops dripped from the leaves and washed the tears from my face. I ran. Along the river, clouds hovered low to the ground. I remembered what Chuck told me about how he prayed while he ran.

I raised both hands while I continued to run and said, "God, please help my grandson."

My words returned from the clouds a few feet above me.

I looked at the swirling mist. No one was there. I shouted, "God, please help Landon."

Had my prayer bounced off the clouds? "Why don't you hear me, God?"

A thought entered my mind. It was so loud I thought I had

heard a voice through the clouds. "It's the sin."

Again, I looked around. Where did that come from? Whose sin? What sin? The thought lingered in my head and bounced around like an echo. "It's the sin."

Wet, I shivered, lowered my hands, and walked home.

That night I struggled to fall asleep. When I did, I slept a couple of hours then woke with the same words in my head, "It's the sin." The words haunted me. Had I lost my mind?

I tossed and turned until daybreak—time to go to work.

Before I did, I opened the door to Mom's room then walked to her bedside. She was awake. "Good morning," I said and smiled at her. "Kathy will be in with your breakfast in a few minutes."

She looked at me, didn't speak, then looked at her old Bible on the nightstand beside her bed.

I reached for the book, and it fell open in my hands. I thumbed through a few pages then stopped on Isaiah 59. I read verses one and two silently.

Wow, I thought, this is it. I reread verse two, this time out loud, "But your iniquities have separated between you and your God, and your sins have hid his face from you, that he will not hear." (Isaiah 59:2 KJV)

I closed the Bible. Mom smiled. I tucked the book under my arm and carried it to my shop.

That day, I couldn't keep my mind on the task at hand and didn't get much work done. Instead, I read Mom's Bible.

After work, I laced my running shoes and hit the trail again. Clouds still shrouded the mountains. Colder air invaded. I tried to stay warm by running harder than usual through the wet fields and misty forest. When I arrived at the place along the river, we call the big swimming hole, I fell to my knees on a rock outcropping at the edge of the water, raised my hands, shivered, and prayed, "My sins have separated us. Please forgive me. I have read how Jesus died for my sins. I accept the gift of Christ and ask You to come into my life."

I fell forward on the rock. Tears streamed from my cheeks. "Please hear my prayers. Please help my grandson."

There was no echo. I raised my head and wiped my eyes as the sky became brighter. Warmth wrapped around me like a blanket, and I stopped shivering. I felt a shift, a change in everything. I knew, no matter what happened, Landon would be okay, and so would I.

Chapter 26

Highs and Lows

On the last day of March 2011, our business phone rang. A cheerful recorded voice of a young lady spoke. I thought, telemarketer, and almost hung up. My ears perked when the girl said, "Landon Joines." I sat in our desk chair and listened.

"The students at Sparta Elementary School are conducting a diaper drive for Landon Joines."

My jaw dropped. God had motivated children to help my grandson with his diaper rash problem. My eyes teared. Keeping Landon in diapers created a financial burden for our family. He used thirty to forty each day—four times the average. We couldn't go anywhere with Landon without bringing eight or ten diapers. Most evenings, if Shelly didn't purchase a box or two on her way home from work, I did. Because the IRS didn't consider diapers a transplant-related expense, we couldn't use donated funds. The money came from Jeremiah's family budget or ours.

God knew of our need. I raised my head. "Thank you."

A couple of mornings later, I drove Ezekiel, who now attended Sparta Elementary, to school. As we waited in the drop-off line, Ezekiel started to squirm. "Why is this line moving slow? I'm going to be late."

When we neared the front of the line, a girl jumped from a vehicle and ran toward the entrance. Then a child from another car did the same. And another. Most carried large boxes of diapers.

We reached the entrance, Ezekiel jumped out, and as I drove past the school parking lot, and a group of students carrying boxes of diapers from vehicles, I swallowed hard and whispered a prayer, "Thank You."

Two weeks later, our family joined the students in the school cafeteria to count the mountain of diaper boxes. It was more than six feet high and twelve feet wide. We celebrated as the students counted 10,000 diapers, enough to last my grandson almost a year. I smiled and snapped pictures.

Landon ran to the pile. He laughed and giggled while he climbed. The students cheered when my grandson reached the top and sat on a box, like a king. Shelly stood close by to make sure he didn't fall off his throne. He joined the class that brought in the most diapers for a romp in a bouncy house a local business donated. Afterward, he and the students ate cake and ice cream. When the party ended, we loaded the diapers in my enclosed trailer. I hauled them to my shop and stored them. No more evening stops at stores to buy diapers.

The next Saturday, we celebrated Landon's second birthday with a family meal at our home. Then, while Ezekiel, Gavin, and Braiden jumped on a trampoline in our back yard, Jeremiah and I walked with Landon along the river behind the house. Jeremiah knelt beside his son and skipped a rock across the water. Landon threw one and laughed when it landed with a plop. My heart filled with love as I watched my son play with his son.

Because Shelly worked at the restaurant and bowling alley, when Landon wasn't in the hospital, Jeremiah had become Landon's primary caregiver. We didn't trust his care to anyone else, and insurance wouldn't have paid for it anyway. I don't think anyone, even a registered nurse, could have provided more compassionate or better care. I've often thought that my son and daughter-in-law should have received a nursing degree for the skills they acquired and the experience they gained while caring for their son.

Landon tossed rocks until he was tired. Despite Jeremiah's back problems, he placed Landon on his shoulders and carried him back home.

Shelly corralled everyone around Landon, who wore a paper party hat and sat in a high chair at one end of our dining room table. The birthday boy stared wide-eyed at a custom-baked cake, made from two dozen individually wrapped cupcakes. He pointed at the flickering flame atop the number two, and his face glowed. I focused on the candle—two. It was the magic number, the age the Boston transplant doctor said Landon should reach before a transplant. He made it. My throat tightened, and I couldn't get the words out to help my family when they sang happy birthday.

Landon took a deep breath. The older boys leaned in. Then all blew the flame from the candle. Landon squealed, laughed, and rubbed his hands together.

Shelly pulled the cupcakes apart. I reached for one.

Kathy slapped my hand. "Too many points." Her eyes gleamed.

"I'll run an extra mile." I grinned, then took a big bite, smearing white and green icing on my mustache in the process.

Kathy laughed.

In the first four months of 2011, Kathy lost thirty-five pounds. I shed forty-five. My wife rewarded herself with much needed new clothes, and I registered for the New River Half Marathon.

May 7, I raised both fists in the air when I crossed the finish line for the 13.1-mile run, finishing in two hours and five minutes. Two hours later, when Chuck finished the whole marathon—26.2 miles—I called and congratulated him.

That evening Kathy and I sat in rocking chairs on our front porch. We watched Landon play in the yard. Adrenaline still coursed through my veins while I babbled about how much I enjoyed the run. After a while, I shared a thought. "I wonder if I could run the Grandfather Mountain Marathon."

A few days earlier, I read an article in a running magazine where the author rated Grandfather as one of the toughest marathons in America.

Kathy shook her head. "You're fifty-four-years-old, a runner for less than six months, and you don't have enough time to train. Besides, people die running marathons."

I looked at the ground. "You're right. It's too dangerous. I should use my time to work on another fundraiser, not to train for a marathon."

Our little grandson pushed a plastic toy lawnmower across the yard in front of us.

The gears in my mind turned. "Runners raise funds for charities all the time." I smiled. "What if I ask people to donate a dollar a mile and run the marathon to raise money for Landon's transplant?"

Kathy shook her head again and rose from the rocking chair. She knew what made me tick. Grandfather Mountain presented a challenge I couldn't resist. She pointed her finger at me, "You better not die doing it," then walked into the house.

I called the most experienced marathon runner I knew, Chuck.

At first, his tone sounded skeptical. "Grandfather Mountain is a hard marathon for anyone." He spoke from experience, having run Grandfather Mountain fifteen times. Then, his words softened, "Knowing you as I do, if you stick to a strict training schedule, I think you can run it."

With Chuck's advice, I developed a plan—long runs on the weekends, followed by short runs during the week, culminating with a twenty-mile run two weeks before the race. With a plan in place to train for the marathon, eight weeks away, I needed to figure out how to raise money.

If I convinced thirty-eight people to donate one-dollar per mile—$26.20—I would raise $1000 if I finished the race. Two days after I posted my plan for the fundraiser on Landon's website, the pledges surpassed my goal. Now, I could justify running the marathon by helping my grandson at the same time.

On May 22, almost three months after he recovered from the flu, Landon's temperature rose again. The transplant doctor suspected bacterial infection and admitted him to the hospital. She guessed right. Although not Klebsiella, but still a dangerous staph bacteria. At Duke, the nurses administered more antibiotics. Landon fought to beat the infection and keep his central line.

While he did, most evenings, I ran on the back roads in our rural community and prayed for my grandson. I told God about my fears and desires while I clicked off the miles.

In the mornings, before I went to work, I read from a Bible. I talked to God when I prayed, and God spoke to me when I read the Bible. Most mornings, I found a passage of scripture related to what I prayed about the evening before. I prayed for Landon, then read how Jesus blessed children, "And he took them up in in his arms, put his hands upon them, and blessed them." (Mark 10:16 KJV)

I prayed again, "Jesus, bless my grandson."

Landon needed all the help he could get to fight this infection. He struggled with the unseen enemy and lashed out at those he could see—the nurses and his parents. On the second night in the hospital, he cried and screamed for hours. His parents couldn't calm him. Finally, a nurse gave him a sedative, and he fell asleep.

When he did, his exhausted parents collapsed into recliners and slept too.

A week later, Landon's temperature returned to normal, and he didn't lose his central line. Although he won the battle, the victory came at a cost. He returned home in a weakened state. More so than after his fight with the flu. When awake, he wanted his grandmother and stayed close to her, often while Kathy cared for Mom at the same time.

While my wife stood by the bed and spoon-fed Mom pureed vegetables, I helped Landon drag a laundry basket full of stuffed animals into Mom's room. Landon tossed a dozen of his furry friends onto the bed. I helped him climb. Kathy and I raised and latched the metal rails on each side of the hospital bed so Landon couldn't tumble off.

Mom, stone-faced, watched Landon. Her lips now drooped in a permanent, involuntary frown. She was unable to speak. A vehicle horn beeped in the driveway, and Shelly retrieved a package, too big for our mailbox, from the postwoman. She brought the box to Mom's room and opened it. Inside she found a note from Whitney, the photographer.

Whitney's friend, Rebekah, from Charlotte, had knitted a prayer shawl for Landon. Shelly pulled the fluffy blue shawl from the package, held it close to her face, then tossed it onto Mom's bed. Landon surrounded himself, and his great grandmother with stuffed animals, then pulled the shawl over the sheets on my mother's hips, laid his head on it, closed his eyes, and sucked his green pacifier.

"Oh, how sweet," Shelly said.

Tears filled my eyes as I watched Landon, who fought for his life, together with his great-grandmother nearing the end of hers.

I thought of my long-deceased Appalachian grandmother; we called her Granny. She would have described Landon as a "frail young'un." In her time, frail young'uns didn't survive. I feared that without a transplant, soon, the next infection or virus would kill him.

Chapter 27

The Transplant

The call came a few minutes before 2:00 p.m. on June 16, 2011.

Standing on the back porch of the small house, Jeremiah pulled the phone away from his ear, placed his hand over the mouthpiece, and shouted, "We have an organ. It's a perfect match." Thirty feet away, Kathy held Landon while he sat on the edge of a trampoline in our yard. Shelly and I watched from a sidewalk in-between. My heart leapt into my throat.

"There's one problem," my son said, still holding the phone in his hand. "The leader of the transplant team is out of town. If we accept this organ, her assistant will lead the team."

For several seconds, the four of us stared at each other in silence. Kathy bit her lower lip, Shelly held her breath, while Jeremiah seemed frozen on the steps. I swallowed hard. If complications arose during the surgery, or if Landon's body rejected the graft, he would die. After ten months on the transplant list, if we turned down this organ, we might not find another in time to save his life. We had prayed for a transplant. God help us make this life or death decision.

On the phone, the transplant coordinator waited for an answer.

We trusted the team. Duke hired the best. In unison, the four of us said, "Yes."

Kathy placed a hand over her mouth. Shelly's eyes teared. Jeremiah told the coordinator of our decision. I raised both hands in the air. "Thank you, God."

This was it. Twenty-six months of fighting to keep Landon alive long enough to get a transplant were over.

The coordinator told Jeremiah not to race to the hospital, because the organ wouldn't arrive for several hours, but get there.

We didn't rush around or throw suitcases in the van as we had for a previous call. Our hearts beat fast, but we moved slow. Actions seemed rehearsed. They were. During the past ten months, this scene played out in our minds hundreds of times.

I called my sister, asked her to come to stay with Mom, then packed a big suitcase for Kathy and me, and loaded it in the trunk of our car. Jessica, who was in our house with Mom when the call came, agreed to remain until my sister arrived and to care for Ezekiel.

Kathy continued to stand by our grandson at the trampoline.

"I want him to play for as long as he can," she said.

He did. Oblivious to the event unfolding, he bounced and laughed with cousins Gavin and Braiden.

Jeremiah placed two suitcases in their van, along with an unopened box of diapers, then pulled the rear hatch shut. I stood beside the vehicle and looked at my son. My throat tightened. I turned away, fearing if we made eye contact, we'd both start bawling.

Shelly carried a diaper bag to the vehicle and opened the sliding door.

When Jeremiah strapped Landon in his car seat, Jessica kissed her nephew then sobbed. We couldn't hold back any longer. Kathy lost it. We all did.

We hugged each other and whispered, "He'll be okay."

Not wanting to frighten Landon, who sucked on his pacifier and looked puzzled, Jeremiah closed the sliding door. I wrapped my arm around my wife, led her to our vehicle, and waved good-bye to Jessica and the older boys.

We descended the mountain behind Jeremiah's van. Kathy dabbed runny mascara with a tissue. I placed my hand on her forearm but didn't speak.

Questions and possible outcomes swirled through my mind. Would my grandson survive the marathon surgery? Would his body accept or reject the transplant?

We followed our son's vehicle while he weaved through rush-hour traffic. Kathy opened a water bottle. Feeling sick, I sipped. At 5:45 p.m., two-and-one-half hours after leaving home, our two cars pulled into the parking deck at Duke University Medical Center.

I stepped out of the car, stretched, and looked across the street. There it was, the hospital where they would save my grandson's life. I breathed deep and tried to swallow the lump in my throat.

In the lobby, Jeremiah and Shelly checked in at the admission window. Landon ran to the fountain. He leaned over the side, pointed at the mound of coins under the gurgling water, looked at me, and smiled. Remembering an earlier visit to the fountain, I nodded and smiled back.

A male transport nurse arrived with a wheelchair, but Landon didn't want to ride. He shook his head, reached for his parents' hands, and pulled them toward the elevators. He seemed eager to get to his room.

There, Shelly and two nurses got him settled. He laid his head on his pillow. Shelly unpacked his bag of toys and placed his pacifiers—all five, orange, blue, green, purple, and pink—on the sheet beside him. I chuckled when Landon exchanged one pacifier for another while he watched cartoons. Did my grandson notice the difference between this admission and his previous stays? He wasn't sick this time, and the nurses hadn't stuck him with any needles. Did he rotate between the different colored pacifiers to deal with the anxiety?

I walked into the hall and looked in both directions. Nothing. No signs of a surgical team coming to get Landon. I returned to the room. Ten minutes later, I looked again, then again — still nothing.

Two hours after we arrived, Kathy choked up. She walked into the hall. I followed.

"Why haven't they come to get Landon yet?" she trembled.

I shook my head. Not knowing the answer, I wrapped my arms around my wife.

About 8:00 p.m., Jeremiah and I went to the cafeteria for a sandwich and coffee. On the way back to Landon's room, we walked by the nurses' station. Jeremiah recognized one from the transplant team, and he asked if the organ had arrived. She pursed her lips and slowly shook her head.

I stiffened when I realized what was happening.

We weren't just waiting for the organ. We were waiting for the child to die.

I lowered my head and closed my eyes—that poor family.

After Jeremiah finished talking with the nurse, I said to him, "Go on without me. I'll be there in a few minutes."

I moseyed outside and sat on a bench in front of the hospital. For a few moments, I didn't focus on my anxiety—our anxiety—to get Landon into the operating room. Instead, I thought of the parents and grandparents of the child about to die. And the gaping hole in their hearts that the child would leave behind. Grateful for their decision to donate organs, I leaned forward, buried my face in my hands, and whispered, "Thank you."

When I returned to the room, Landon stood in his bed, raised his shirt, and pointed at the marks on his belly the surgeon made while I was gone. Shelly tickled his stomach. He giggled and sat back in the bed.

I stroked his hair and smiled.

Jeremiah sat in a chair and stared out the window at the fading light. A moment later, Landon, with his orange pacifier in his mouth, crawled into his lap and laid his head on his dad's chest. Jeremiah's chin quivered. He wrapped his arms around his son and rocked.

My son, my grandson, our family had endured so much since Landon's birth.

While we waited, Kathy posted to social media, and I streamed video from the hospital room to our friends and family.

At 10:30 p.m., a nurse gave Landon a sedative. Shelly and Kathy crawled in bed and lay on each side of him. His mother held his hand, and his grandmother stroked his soft curls. Sniffling, I snapped pictures while he drifted off to sleep.

I looked at my phone—Midnight. More than six hours after our arrival, I was still anxious. I sat in a chair and shut my eyes but couldn't sleep.

Finally, a little after 1:00 a.m., four nurses and an assistant surgeon from the transplant team entered Landon's room. Their glowing faces radiated positive energy, but their sudden presence seemed to suck the air out of the room. I stood and gasped. Kathy, Jeremiah, and Shelly did the same.

A nurse removed the IV fluids from a stand and laid the bag

in Landon's bed beside his pillow.

"Wait," I said. "Let us pray for my grandson before you take him away."

We circled Landon's bed, each of us with a different visceral reaction—Shelly sniffled, Jeremiah gritted his teeth, Kathy shook.

Again, I struggled to breathe and sobbed, "God, please take care of Landon. Guide the hands of the surgeons."

Jeremiah caught Shelly when her knees buckled.

We moved aside. The team unlocked the wheels on the bed and rolled it into the hall with us a few steps behind.

At the entrance to the operating room, I placed my hand on Kathy's back. She kissed our grandson. I held her in my arms while the team rolled him through the doors with Jeremiah and Shelly following. Kathy and I stayed behind. We weren't allowed.

Weak and shaky, we stood at the closed door and held each other until strong enough to walk to the empty waiting room. I never imagined it would be so hard to let go of our grandson, to trust the transplant team. And God. I wish I could say my newfound faith didn't waver. But I trembled with fear for my grandson.

A few minutes before 3:00 a.m., Jeremiah entered the waiting room. He sat beside me, leaned back, and stretched. "The surgery hasn't started yet."

My mouth dropped open.

Jeremiah said, "We're still waiting for the organ." He rubbed his eyes, stood, and returned to the pre-op room.

What was taking so long? I leaned back and placed my hands on my head. The surgeons wouldn't have taken Landon to the operating room unless the donor had died, but they would delay the surgery until the organ was on the way. Somewhere, in another hospital, another team of surgeons was operating on the donor. I wanted to know more, but confidentiality laws prevented the transplant team from telling us anything about the intestine or the donor.

My heart still hurt for the family. How old? Why? I guess all that mattered is a part of their child would live on and save my grandson's life.

At 5:00 a.m. Kathy woke from dozing on my shoulder. "Is it here yet?"

"No," I said. "It's on the way. The transplant team is operating on Landon now."

Kathy covered her mouth with her hand, stifled her sobs, and laid her head back on my shoulder.

Jeremiah and Shelly came from the pre-op room and sat across from us. Shelly shivered and stared at a wall. Jeremiah, his face ghostlike, tapped his foot on the floor and his fingers on the arm of the chair.

Exhausted, I couldn't help but doze.

My son nudged my shoulder around 7:00 a.m. "The intestine is almost here."

While other families of surgery patients trickled into the waiting room, I stumbled half-awake to the restroom. After splashing water on my face, I went to the cafeteria for coffee. I don't know the exact time, but I think the organ arrived around 9:00 a.m. Five more hours of surgery followed.

At 2:00 p.m., the surgeon opened the door to the waiting room and stepped in. Her smile lit the room, and I knew that he made it. I jumped to my feet and helped Kathy to hers. The four of us rushed toward the surgeon. She motioned us to a small conference room.

You couldn't have slapped the smile off my face. The surgery went as planned. Perfect. No problems.

We sat and faced the surgeon.

Her face morphed into one of concern. "It's not over."

I bit my lip.

"A lot of things can still go wrong," she said. "Landon should begin to wake in a couple of hours. He'll be in a lot of pain. We'll keep him as comfortable as we can and watch for complications. You can see Landon, but only two at a time in the recovery room."

I smiled, and we hugged the surgeon.

Jeremiah and Shelly hurried to the recovery room. Kathy lowered her head.

I wrapped my arm around her while we walked back to the waiting room. "We'll see our grandson soon."

She nodded and wiped her eyes with her fingertips.

In the waiting room, I posted to the blog: "The Transplant

is Done!" Responses flooded in. Most said they would pray and asked how else they could help. I wrote, "Pledge to the marathon." Within minutes pledges poured in.

Sometime in the mid-afternoon, Jeremiah came to the waiting room. Kathy, excited and shaking, joined Shelly in the recovery room.

Jeremiah sat across from me and leaned his head back.

I smiled at my strong yet tired son. He and Shelly had done all they could do to get Landon to this point. Now, their son had a chance. And that's all any of us could ask for—a chance.

I lowered my head. "God, give Jeremiah and Shelly the strength to continue. And heal Landon."

An hour later, the nurses moved Landon to an intensive care unit. After a quick discussion, and at my insistence, Jeremiah and Shelly went to the cafeteria. I hurried to join my wife and grandson.

The sight of Landon in the ICU made me gasp. I swallowed hard and held my breath. The tubes. The wires. The colostomy bag and bandages. A nurse stood on the left side of the bed and looked at a monitor. Kathy sat on the right and rubbed Landon's forehead. Then he moved, and I finally exhaled.

"He's waking," Kathy said.

His chin quivered. So did mine. He grimaced, but his eyes remained closed. He rolled his head toward his grandmother's voice as far as the tubes in his mouth and nose allowed.

An alarm beeped fast.

I covered my mouth.

The nurse said, "Rapid heartbeat. Time for more pain meds."

After she administered the medication, Landon's heart slowed, and he slept.

Still tense, I stared at my grandson.

Soon, my respirations matched the hypnotic sound of the ventilator. I couldn't stop myself. With each swoosh, I took a breath then exhaled.

Come on, Landon. You're strong. You can do this.

The spell broke when an hour later, he thrashed and gagged until the nurse removed the vent tube. Then he cried in a high-pitched raspy voice. The alarm beeped again. The nurse administered more pain meds.

A few minutes later, Jeremiah and Shelly returned from the cafeteria. Their son was quiet. A nurse told them they should go to the hotel and get some sleep while Kathy and I stayed with Landon.

"You'll need the rest," the nurse said. "Tomorrow will be a rough day."

Chapter 28

Duke Chapel and Recovery

The night following the transplant, the nurses kept Landon sedated. In the dim ICU, they watched monitors, checked his temperature, and listened to his lungs. He woke a couple of times and moaned. When he did, a nurse gave him more medication while Kathy caressed his forehead until he fell asleep.

A little after 2:00 a.m., Jeremiah and Shelly, having rested a few hours, returned to the hospital. Kathy and I walked to the hotel and crawled into bed.

At 8:00 a.m., Saturday, I woke refreshed and called the hospital.

"He's sitting in bed, wrapped in his prayer shawl, watching *Toy Story*," Jeremiah said.

It seemed impossible. I left my grandson a few hours earlier, still asleep or moaning in pain. How could he now be awake and watching a video?

"That's great news," I said. "I'll come to the hospital when I get back from my run."

My training plan called for a long run on this date, but not in Durham. While I laced my running shoes, I read some of the messages and prayers flooding Landon's website. Tears blurred my vision. Overnight, pledges for the marathon doubled to $2,000, twice my goal. Encouraged, I hit the sidewalk running.

The clear blue sky over the campus of Duke University beckoned me to run fast and praise God. I did both. Red and white azaleas bloomed along the walkways. The aroma of southern pines filled my nostrils, and warm air filled my lungs. My spirit soared.

I ran across Cameron Boulevard and into Duke Forest. Two hours on the loop trail gave me the miles I needed. Back on the campus streets, I spotted the Gothic spires of Duke Chapel. My route didn't call for me to go to the Chapel, yet I felt drawn.

I walked around the massive stone cathedral and sipped from my water bottle. The architecture and landscape created a medieval atmosphere. At the thick wooden doors to the sanctuary, I grabbed the wrought iron ring and pulled. The door opened. Behind it was another wooden door. I pushed, and it opened.

"Hello." My voice echoed.

No one answered. I stepped in and shut the door. The cold air inside chilled my sweat-soaked shirt. I shivered. Dim lights above the nave illuminated stone arches on the sides of the sanctuary. A beam of light through stained glass brightened the alter. I walked forward a few steps, rubbing my left palm over the top of the wooden pews, then stopped and listened. Nothing except the sound of my footsteps reverberated in the empty church. I continued forward.

At the marble altar, I knelt. Everything leading to Landon's transplant had fallen into place. I had feared that even if I learned about intestinal transplants, talked to the right doctors, and gave my son and daughter-in-law the best advice, my grandson would die anyway. He hadn't.

"Thank you, Jesus," I said weeping.

A warmth reminiscent of my time at the river surrounded me. I lay on the altar and promised God I would share the story of how He saved my grandson—the miracle. Comforted by the presence I felt, I remained at the Chapel until a strong desire to see Landon pulled me away.

My legs wobbled while I jogged back to the hotel. I showered, dressed, and, with renewed energy, rushed to the hospital. I expected to see my grandson as Jeremiah had described him, sitting and watching a video. Instead, I stopped when I entered the room.

A nurse stood on the right side of Landon's bed. She systematically patted his back between his shoulder blades while he cried, "I sorry, I sorry."

I grabbed Kathy's arm and pointed at the nurse, "What's she doing?"

She shook her head. Tears dripped from her cheeks. "He has congestion in his lungs. They've got to break it loose, or he'll get pneumonia."

Tense, I swallowed hard and bit my lower lip.

Shelly leaned on the left side of the bed with one hand on the back of Landon's head, the other on his bottom propping her son on his side so the nurse could continue. Tears filled Shelly's eyes. Jeremiah stared out a window with his fist clenched. At the foot of the bed, another yellow smiley face balloon floated. The mouth should have turned down instead of up.

Landon continued to cry, "I sorry, I sorry."

A long minute later, the nurse stopped. She and Shelly eased Landon to his back. He whimpered. The nurse stroked his forehead, lowered her head, and left the room.

Shelly sniffled and rubbed Landon's lips with the tip of his green pacifier. He opened his mouth and sucked it in. I breathed deep and wiped my eyes while Jeremiah plopped into a chair and closed his. Kathy pulled a white sheet up to Landon's chin, then kissed his cheek.

In the early afternoon, Landon's oxygen levels dropped to dangerous levels. Hoping to avoid a return to the ventilator, the nurse beat on his back more and encouraged him to cough. I couldn't bear to watch again, so when she did, I left the room and walked down the hall far enough that I could no longer hear Landon's cry, "I sorry."

The respiratory exercises continued hourly until the phlegm broke loose. That evening, Landon coughed and gagged. Jeremiah rolled him on his side and rubbed his back while Shelly held a paper towel under his mouth and whispered, "Cough Landon, cough. Come on. You can do it."

He did but cried between the coughs and gags. Soon, he breathed easier. His oxygen levels rose.

Late in the night, his condition improved enough that Jeremiah and Shelly felt comfortable in leaving. They went to the hotel while Kathy and I stayed another night with our grandson.

The next morning, Sunday, church congregations all over western North Carolina prayed for Landon. While they did, two nurses helped my grandson get out of bed and on his feet. The nurses held his hands and encouraged him to walk around the ICU. He winced with each movement yet took several steps. One of the nurses told us, the more he walks, the faster he will recover, and the less likely the congestion will return to his lungs. He got out of bed a couple more times during the day and walked a few more steps each time.

During the afternoon, the surgeon listened to Landon's belly with a stethoscope. She smiled. "It's alive. Juices are flowing."

I also smiled, knowing we did the right thing by pushing to get Landon a transplant before his liver failed, and he became too sick to survive. He was strong.

That evening, Kathy and I didn't want to leave Durham, but we didn't have much choice. My sister couldn't stay with Mom any longer, and I needed to open our business, get back to work, and pay bills. We smothered Landon with kisses, Jeremiah and Shelly with hugs, then returned home.

On the third day of recovery, the nurses moved Landon to a "step down room" on the pediatric ward. There, an assigned nurse continued to monitor him.

The hall made a big loop that passed by the nurses' station. With the help of his parents, he walked the loop. Each time he did, he passed the nurses' station, where the nurses cheered and gave him a ticket that he could exchange for a toy. The more tickets he earned, the better the item he received.

When Landon's transplant surgeon made her rounds, she joined him in the hall for a short walk. She smiled and held his hand. He looked at her and grinned behind his pacifier. Landon walked four loops by evening then redeemed his tickets for a coloring book and stickers of *Toy Story* and Mickey Mouse.

In the days that followed, he continued to heal. The nurses moved him to a regular room, where he placed stickers on everything within his reach, the bed, the tables, and the monitors. Get well cards, balloons, and stuffed animals arrived daily. Shelly taped the cards on the walls, tied the balloons to the bed, and surrounded Landon with stuffed animals and toys—a Mister Potato Head and plastic colorful building blocks.

The doctors conducted numerous tests, which included a biopsy to check for rejection, and tests to monitor the levels of the anti-rejection medicine. The test results looked good. The nurses introduced fluids through Landon's G-tube. Again, the plumbing worked.

A week after the surgery, the transplant doctor removed the staples.

With my grandson recovering, my thoughts turned to finances. Barring any problems, Landon would get out of the hospital in a few weeks. However, the doctors wouldn't allow him to leave Durham for months, so the family would need an apartment near the hospital. We had raised more than $25,000, but how long could it last? We didn't know how long Landon and his family would need to stay in Durham.

A week after the transplant, I checked the marathon page on Landon's web site. The pledges approached $4,500. More came in daily. With the marathon two weeks away, I continued to train on the back roads of our community. I ran most days and prayed every day.

In the hospital, there was no sign of rejection. There were a few setbacks, scares, and delays. Like when he developed a mystery fever that lasted three days, and we never discovered the reason for it. Nothing major. Landon fought and grew stronger. God continued to bless him.

By the day of the marathon, the pledges topped $12,000— beyond my wildest dreams. However, doubt crept into my mind. I had stuck to my training schedule except for one run, the twenty-miler, the most important. After Landon's transplant, because we drove to Durham on the weekends, I couldn't make time for the longest run. Without the twenty-miler, and the experience I would have gained, could I still run 26.2 miles from Boone to Grandfather Mountain and collect the money to support my grandson's recovery?

God, help me.

Chapter 29

The Grandfather Mountain Marathon

I trembled and stumbled from our car in the parking lot at Kidd Brewer Stadium, on the campus of Appalachian State University, July 9, 2011, in Boone, North Carolina. With both hands atop the vehicle, I pretended to stretch my calves, hoping the other runners hadn't noticed my nervousness.

A runner for a short seven months, I felt like a fraud—an amateur among elites. What made me think I could run a marathon anyway, and one of the toughest marathons in America at that? But here I was, having announced my intentions to the world; and determined to collect the money to support Landon's recovery, I couldn't back out now. The thought and the cold air made me shiver.

Although forecasters predicted a warm day, it didn't start that way. The flimsy running shorts and shirt I wore didn't protect me from the morning chill. Soft blue light bathed the mountains while mist rose from the hollers. My teeth chattered. I placed my long-billed runner's hat on my head and jogged in place to get warm.

Wearing a sweater over her shoulders, Kathy held a pink cowbell close to her chest. Our grandson Gavin was with us. He retrieved my grey running belt from the trunk of the car.

The belt held four plastic flasks, each containing ten ounces of pre-mixed orange energy drink. I placed an energy bar and a wad of toilet paper in a zippered pouch on the belt then strapped it onto my waist. I planned to begin nibbling on the energy bar at the halfway point and hoped I wouldn't need the toilet paper.

From the stands inside the stadium, we searched for Chuck among the mass of runners on the track. We spotted him in the middle of the crowd, about twenty yards behind the starting line, and waved until we got his attention. I kissed Kathy, hugged Gavin, then ran down the steps and joined Chuck.

He grabbed my hands. "Let's pray," he said, his voice as nervous as mine.

We did. In the middle of several hundred runners, we prayed for a safe run and God's help.

A starter pointed a pistol in the air and fired; we surged forward. The forty-fourth Grandfather Mountain Marathon began. My first. Chuck's sixteenth.

Kathy rang her cowbell and shouted, "Woohoo. Go, Eldon. Go, Chuck," while Gavin took video with my camera.

The two would catch a bus to Grandfather Mountain and meet

me at the track at MacRae Meadows, the finish line. I set a goal to get there in five hours or less. Organizers held the marathon in conjunction with the Southern Scottish Highland Games, which were underway on the Mountain. To make room for the other events, the officials closed the track to runners after five hours into the marathon and gave those who arrived late medals but wouldn't let them finish on the track. I wanted to finish on the track.

A few runners wore tartan kilts. Even though the morning started cool, several men ran without shirts.

I felt uncomfortable with the fast pace of the crowd, yet I had no choice but to stay with the pack or get run over. We ran around the track, then exited the stadium and headed down the hill toward Rivers Street. I sucked in the fresh air. My heart rate surged.

"Pace yourself," Chuck said, while we ran beside each other. "We've started too fast."

We slowed and allowed several runners to pass. Then my competitive nature took hold, and I sped up.

Chuck bumped his shoulder against mine. "It's not how fast you are at the beginning, but how strong you are at the end that determines if you'll survive."

I thought about Landon. Even though he was weakened by the obstacles he overcame, at the end of the long journey, Landon was strong enough to survive the transplant. I slowed and let more runners pass.

The police blocked traffic on Highway 321, a busy four-lane road through the commercial section of Boone. We turned south and ran by the fast-food restaurants and shopping centers before turning west on a side road that led out of town and into the higher mountains.

Having run the mountain many times, Chuck knew the route better than anyone else. Before we left town, he veered into a fenced parking lot and behind a big truck for a pee stop. He urged me to do the same. "There aren't any good places for several miles."

I didn't feel the need, even though I drank a thirty-two-ounce Gatorade before the run started, so I didn't. A bad decision.

Chuck caught up with me at the bottom of the first big hill on the outskirts of Boone. "Walk," he said.

"What do you mean, walk? We've only run a couple of miles. I've got plenty of energy."

"These first hills leading into the mountains are steep but short. You can walk them almost as fast as you can run them. If you run them, you'll regret it on Highway 221."

Highway 221—the last nine miles of the run to Grandfather Mountain, almost all uphill.

We walked the first hill out of Boone, while most runners passed us.

"We'll catch them later," Chuck said with a wink.

A camaraderie existed between Chuck and other alumni of Grandfather Mountain. Several walked with us and laughed while they told stories from previous marathons.

I pulled a flask from my belt and squeezed a couple of ounces of sweet orange liquid into my mouth. Chuck didn't bring anything to drink. I offered him some.

He shook his head and pointed at the road. "There's an aid station at the top of the hill."

When we reached it, he grabbed two paper cups of water, eight ounces, from a volunteer, and drank both. We ran again until we reached the next steep hill, then walked. This continued for five miles. Hill after hill, we climbed. When we walked, I sipped the energy drink. We passed another aid station. Again, Chuck drank water.

Soon, the urge to pee hit me hard. The steep road banks and houses didn't provide a place to get off the road and go, so I held it. When the pain became unbearable, and I didn't think I could hold it any longer, we passed a house, ran around a curve, and the forest leveled out. I ran into the laurel bushes and behind a tree. Out of sight of the other runners, I relieved myself. Chuck took a pee break also. We emerged from the trees at the same time.

I naturally ran at a slower pace than Chuck. I had held him back and felt bad about that. I appreciated him hanging with me, but I didn't want to slow him to the point that he couldn't finish in less than five hours.

"Go on without me, Chuck. I've got this," I said.

"Are you sure? I'll stay if you want me to."

"I'm sure," I said, a half-truth. The whole truth was, finish or not, I needed to do this on my own.

Chuck understood and nodded.

Before he left, he rattled off a slew of advice. He told me about two more steep hills that I should walk, one after exiting the Parkway and crossing under a bridge, the other near the end of a gravel road which he said wasn't much more than a driveway leading to Highway 221.

"Save your energy for 221," he said again. "You'll need it." He turned to leave, then turned back. "Go easy on the orange drink. It'll make you sick. Drink water."

A few minutes later, Chuck pulled ahead, then disappeared around a curve, into the swirling mist on the narrow mountain road. Fog obscured the view and closed in around me.

A few runners ran near me, but we didn't talk or even acknowledge each other. I felt alone. Chuck did what God sent him to do. He gave me all the advice and encouragement he could, but from this point on, finishing was up to me. Could I do it without Chuck beside me? Who would I turn to if something went wrong?

Footsteps approached from behind. A man in a blue plaid kilt and a white T-shirt passed on my right. On the back of his shirt was a stick-figure drawing of a man with a brown beard, long flowing brown hair, and a kilt, who ran. Printed under the stick figure was: "What think ye of Christ?" I smiled and nodded.

A mile later, the sun emerged. The fog turned to steam, the steam to humidity, and the sky cleared. At the crest of a hill, the profile of Grandfather Mountain, which looks more like the profile of Abraham Lincoln, loomed to the south. With a view of the big mountain, I felt a surge of energy and ran faster.

I approached the Parkway, mile eleven, and pumped both fists in the air to celebrate the finish of the steep climb from Boone. A man stepped from the side of the road and snapped my picture. Later, through the Internet, his company would offer to sell me the image. I bought it. I wanted to keep this memory.

At the aid station, I pulled a flask from my belt and sipped orange drink while other runners grabbed paper cups from volunteers.

Most of the route is under the canopy of the forest. So, the first real heat of the day hit me on the two-and-one-half mile, unshaded section, on the Parkway.

The scenic roadway wasn't as steep as the winding backroads that led to it. After a long downhill section that ended at Price Lake, the halfway point in the marathon, I looked at my watch - two hours and sixteen minutes. If I continued at this pace, I could make it to MacRae Meadows in less than five hours. But Highway 221 loomed ahead, the most challenging section, according to Chuck, and every other experienced runner of Grandfather Mountain. My thighs burned. I stared at the road and tried not to think about 221.

I left the Parkway and crossed under the bridge—mile fifteen. Tilting my head back, I gazed at the long steep hill that Chuck warned me about. I walked, nibbled on my energy bar, and sipped the last of the orange drink. From here on, I would depend on the aid stations for water. At the top of the hill, I turned right and ran a mile on a gravel road until it narrowed at a cluster of houses and the bottom of another steep hill.

The sun bore down. The holler trapped heat on both sides and baked me. Sweat soaked every stitch of my clothes and dripped from my nose. A man in a yard sprayed water from a hose into the air for runners to pass through. I did.

At the end of the gravel road, I turned right and stopped. There it was, 221, not a hill, but a mountain. The road ascended for as far as I could see. I pulled the bill of my hat low on my forehead, looked at the pavement ten feet in front of me, and ran. I concentrated on the steady rhythm of my feet. Slow but steady. "Keep moving, keep climbing," I told myself.

Around a curve, a family stood at the end of a driveway handing out sponges soaked in coolers of ice water. I grabbed one, removed my hat, and slapped the icy sponge on top of my head. A cold shock pulsed through my body to the soles of my feet. I rubbed my forehead and cheeks with the sponge and remembered the night we cooled Landon's feverish head.

Refreshed, I felt strong and passed a runner, my first on 221, then another, and another. I ran by a young man who sat on a rock wall rubbing his calves. I recognized him. Earlier that morning, he ran by me on the first big hill out of Boone.

I rounded a curve to the left. In a pullover on the right side of the road, an older woman sat in the passenger seat of a vintage vehicle. My father owned a similar car when I was a child. With the door open toward the road, and her feet on the ground, the woman crocheted. I waved, but the woman didn't respond. I ran by and continued up the mountain. Later, when I asked Chuck about the woman, he didn't remember seeing her.

A mile ahead, while I ran south, a view to the east across the foothills of the Blue Ridge and the Piedmont of North Carolina, opened through the trees. If not for the humidity, I could have seen a hundred miles or more, toward Durham, where Landon walked the halls of the hospital. I smiled. If he could do it, so could I. But at mile twenty-one, my legs burned, and my feet hurt.

While I ran around a hairpin turn to the left with a waterfall on the right, no other runners were near me, yet someone tied bricks to my shoes. At least that's what it felt like. I couldn't raise my feet more than an inch from the road. They skidded along the pavement. My legs wobbled.

What was happening? Was this "The Wall," or what Chuck described as the "Wheels coming off the cart?" Was this the end? If so, I wouldn't finish the marathon and wouldn't collect the money pledged for my grandson.

I raised my hands and looked at the sky. "God, I need you. I can't do this without you. Please help me," I said.

A cool breeze raced off the side of Grandfather Mountain, under the raised portion of the Parkway called the Linn Cove Viaduct, over the waterfall, and me, almost knocking me to the pavement. I filled my lungs with the refreshing air. The weight on my shoes fell away. My feet practically bounced off the pavement.

I ran.

My stride increased. I raised my open hands. "Thank You," I shouted three times.

Sweat still dripped from my nose, chin, and ears. But with renewed energy, I ran faster.

A few minutes later, I spotted a runner in a curve above me. I focused on him and ran until I caught and passed him. Then another runner in another curve, and yet another. They ran slow. Some looked as bad as I had felt a few minutes earlier. A man stumbled from one side of the road to the other.

"Do you need help?" I said when I caught up with him.

He shook his head.

I continued and passed.

Out of orange drink, my mouth dried, and the sweating slowed. A mile later, dehydrated, I ran toward an aid station and the water I craved. When I stopped running, the world turned white and fuzzy.

Kathy's voice filled my head, "Don't die doing it."

Trembling, I grabbed two cups of water and gulped. Then two more. My vision cleared. I ran again and passed two medics who tended to a runner who lay on the side of the road. Someone said, "Cramps."

Not long after I left the aid station, I looked at my running watch, four hours and forty-one minutes. I didn't know how much further to MacRae Meadows, but I had less than twenty minutes to get there and still finish on the track.

A hollow feeling in my gut caused me to hunch forward and droop my shoulders. Nauseated, I ran under a rock bridge, with the Parkway above, and dry heaved. Fearing I couldn't get my legs going again if I stopped, I just ran. I didn't think anymore. Couldn't.

A faint, strange sound drifted from the mountain above me, bagpipes. I rounded a curve. A man stood in the road. He pointed toward a trail. I took it.

Ahead, someone shouted, "Runner coming." A crowd parted to make way. People clapped. I ran up the drive toward MacRae Meadows. The sound of bagpipes grew louder.

Chuck—having finished ten minutes ahead of me—stood with Sherry on a grassy bank to the right of the drive. They clapped and shouted when I ran by.

On the track, a man motioned me to the left. Somewhere in the crowd of spectators, a cowbell rang. Gavin stepped in front of me, then ran beside me. The crowd roared with applause. Bagpipes blared.

Tears, mixed with my sweat, dripped from my cheeks. I raised my hands and crossed the finish line of the Grandfather Mountain Marathon at five hours and two minutes.

"Thank you, Jesus."

Chapter 30

Durham and Death

Within a few weeks of finishing the marathon, I collected all the money pledged. And more. Our total now stood at just under $40,000. I hoped it was enough to support Landon's recovery and any future expenses related to his transplant.

July 19 became a day we had worked toward, dreamed of, and prayed for. Thirty-two days after the transplant, the surgeon finally released Landon from the hospital. On his way out, Landon stopped at the nurses' station and cashed in his tickets for walking laps around the hall—256 tickets representing 128 laps. The nurses took his picture, taped a printed copy to the wall, and declared him the all-time prize winner. They loaded a buggy with new toys as his reward. Landon took his treasure and went to live with his family in a new apartment five miles south of Duke.

The surgeon said, "If he gets sick, get him back to the hospital quick. Things could go bad fast."

Also, the transplant team required Landon to return several times each week for testing, exams, and medication. They monitored his condition to make sure the transplanted intestine worked and watched for any signs of rejection.

With Landon out of the hospital, but still 150 miles away, Kathy learned to use Skype so she could see her grandson. Most days, while she talked with Jeremiah and Shelly, she waved at Landon and said, "Mawmaw loves you." He pointed at the screen, smiled, and waved back. But Skype wasn't enough. We longed to hold our grandson and see for ourselves how he healed. So, each week we visited on Saturdays or Sundays.

The color had returned to Landon's cheeks, and he finally started looking and acting like a normal little boy. With temperatures outside near 100 degrees, we marveled at his energy while he ran around the air-conditioned apartment and played with his toys. Because the central line still provided nutrition and would until proven he could thrive with the new intestine, he wore his backpack or pulled his pump bag behind him. The burden didn't slow him, though.

My heart swelled when, two months after the transplant, my resilient grandson climbed on the sofa, jumped in my lap, and asked me to read a book to him.

One hot Sunday afternoon, Kathy and I lounged around the pool at the apartment complex with Jeremiah and Shelly and watched Roger and Ezekiel swim. Landon wanted to get in the pool, but with the tubes still in his body, he couldn't. Kathy sat on the steps and held him while Landon kicked the water. He cackled when he splashed his grandmother.

In late summer, our weekend visits ended.

Mom's condition grew worse and required Kathy's full attention. She struggled to care for my mother, even to get her to swallow food. The hospice nurses came most days and helped. Mom's doctor offered to insert a feeding tube, but we decided against it. Doing so would prolong the inevitable.

After the marathon, I continued to run several days each week. While I ran, I often prayed for my mother, wife, and grandson.

God had answered my prayers, and those of many others, by healing Landon. He grew stronger, and on October 10, less than four months after the transplant and months sooner than we expected, the transplant team released him to leave Durham.

In the evening, after Jeremiah called with the good news, I stopped by Mom's room before going for a run. "Landon's coming home tomorrow. The transplant is over," I said.

She couldn't respond, yet her eyes told me she understood. During the past several months, atrophy had curled her body into an almost fetal position and contorted her face. I pulled a blanket over her shoulders. Her eyes followed my every move and begged for relief. I swallowed hard, smiled, and backed out of her room.

While I ran, I thought of Mom and her condition. Tears dripped from my cheeks. I raised my arms, "God, my mother is suffering. If it's her time, please take her." I had begged God to keep Landon alive, so how could I now pray for my mother's death? Yet, I couldn't bear to see her suffer longer.

That night, Mom died. Kathy found her in the morning and called me home from a business meeting two hours away. The Hospice nurses delayed the ambulance until I arrived. I stood beside Mom's bed, held Kathy, and struggled to breathe while we sobbed. I believed what Jesus told us, "And if I go and prepare a place for you, I will come again, and receive you unto myself; that where I am, there ye may be also." (John 14:3 KJV)

Mother went to that place. I understood death was a transition, and I would see her again. Still, it hurt to let her go.

But Mom's suffering ended. Her body relaxed, as did her face until it looked like she smiled. She had lived a life of faith and believed long before any of us did that God would save Landon—and me.

And He did.

Chapter 31

Thriving

While Jeremiah and Shelly prepared to leave Durham to come home for Mom's funeral, they discovered Landon's central line was blocked. They went to the hospital, thinking the transplant surgeon would place a new line in Landon's last remaining access site and delay their trip home.

The doctor didn't. She determined that the new intestine could provide the nutrition Landon required, and he no longer needed the line. She removed the last of the lines that for two and one-half years had kept my grandson alive long enough to get a transplant. But several times because of infections, the lines almost killed him. With the line gone, so was the threat of another infection.

Although still grieving Mom's death, I smiled when Jeremiah and Shelly arrived home and told us about the central line. It was another milestone on the road to Landon's recovery.

More than a year later, on October 31, 2012, the surgeons performed an ostomy reversal and removed the bag from Landon's side. Soon after, Landon experienced his first bowel movement. A normal poop. Diarrhea and diaper rash that tortured him before the transplant would not return to hurt him.

A few months later, Landon, almost four years old, bounced into our living room and told us the Make-A-Wish Foundation had granted him a wish. I'm not sure he understood what that meant, but the smiles on Jeremiah and Shelly's faces revealed they did. When Kathy asked Landon what he wanted, he placed his hands on his head to imitate mouse ears, wiggled his fingers, and said, "Mickey, Mickey, Mickey." I think he had been coached.

On March 29, 2013, he and his family traveled to Orlando, Florida. Kathy and I couldn't go but followed via Twitter and frequent phone calls. They stayed a week at the Give Kids the World Village, an 84-acre non-profit resort for children with critical illnesses. The transplant surgeon had given Landon the okay and encouraged him to eat anything he wanted. Landon ate all the pizza and ice cream he could hold. Roger and Ezekiel enjoyed the pool. Jeremiah and Shelly, the rest.

Mickey came to the resort and personally invited Landon to visit The Magic Kingdom. The Disney parks gave Landon the VIP treatment. An escort took him to the front of the line at every ride and allowed him to ride as many times as he wanted. He rode the Haunted Mansion, and It's a Small World more than twenty times each.

Before returning home, they went to the beach for a day.

After the trip, Landon and his family moved to a house in Sparta, about five miles from where Kathy and I lived. In the fall of 2013, two years after the transplant, Landon attended Preschool. A year later, Kindergarten.

As I finished writing this book, eight-and-a-half years after the transplant, Landon, five feet, four inches tall and 108 pounds, attended fifth grade in a public school. Because of his compromised immune system, going to a public school was a big deal. He was educated in a private Christian school until the end of the previous school year when the school closed for financial reasons. Jeremiah and Shelly considered homeschooling but made the difficult decision to place their son in a public school with the hope that Landon could enjoy a normal childhood. That had always been our goal, and now he did. Landon loved his new school and his new friends. And, he didn't get sick.

Other than the scars and the daily rounds of anti-rejection medicine, he was a normal happy boy. He made good grades and displayed his artistic nature by painting, acting, and playing the fiddle. And of course, like all kids his age, my grandson enjoyed video games.

Since the transplant, he has experienced no significant medical problems: no rejection, no infections, and no long hospital admissions.

Kathy and I semi-retired in 2018. Retirement gave us more time to help Jeremiah and Shelly with Landon so they could pursue careers. Jeremiah still has back problems but has learned to live with the pain without surgery or drugs. He works as a project manager for a construction company. Shelly owns a home cleaning service business.

In January 2020, we drove our grandson to Duke for a scheduled clinic visit with the transplant team and an endoscopy to look at the transplanted intestine and do a biopsy. The transplant coordinator smiled while he gave us another excellent report. "All was well," he said.

Late that afternoon, before leaving Durham, we drove to Duke Chapel. Landon, who sat in the back seat, leaned forward. His eyes bulged when the spires of the gothic cathedral came into view through our windshield.

He was still a little groggy from the anesthesia, and Kathy was tired from the long day at the hospital. So, they stayed in the car while I walked to the chapel.

Class was in session at Duke University, and hundreds of students hurried along the sidewalks, rode bicycles on the drives, or stood waiting for buses.

At the chapel, the massive wood doors with the wrought iron rings were open, so I pushed the inner wood doors and entered. Things had changed since my visit on the day after Landon's transplant. A receptionist at a desk told me that after renovations in 2015, the lighting was brighter. She helped me with the terminology for the architecture, which was part of the reason I came. Several other visitors stood admiring the sanctuary and taking pictures.

I thanked the receptionist then walked the long aisle to the front of the church, again brushing the tops of the wooden pews with my left hand. A half dozen people sat scattered in pews, some with heads lowered, others staring at the tall stained glass or the stone ceiling above.

At the altar, with my chin on my chest, I closed my eyes and offered a prayer. A sudden gush of tears surprised me. Years of emotions flowed while I thanked God for continuing to watch over my grandson. I walked back to our car, still wiping my eyes.

"What's wrong?" Kathy said when I climbed into the driver's seat.

"Nothing. Everything is okay."

I pressed *home* on our car's navigation screen, then looked in the rearview mirror and smiled. Landon sang along to a song playing on his cell phone, just like any other kid his age.

To continue following Landon's story and to see numerous pictures of our journey visit: www.landonsstory.com

Acknowledgments

My family and I would like to thank the many churches, people, and organizations that help Landon and us. We encourage readers to support these worthy causes with your finances and or time.

- Brenner Children's Hospital, Wake Forest Baptist Medical Center, Medical Center Boulevard, Winston-Salem, NC 27157

- Ronald McDonald House Winston-Salem, North Carolina; 419 S. Hawthorne Road, Winston-Salem, NC 27103. Phone (336) 723-0228, email info@rmhws.org

- Children's Organ Transplant Association (COTA); 2501 West COTA Drive, Bloomington, IN 47403; Phone (800) 366-2682, email cota@cota.org

- Boston Children's Hospital; Boston Children's Hospital Trust, 401 Park Drive, Suite 602, Boston, MA 02215; Phone (617) 355-6890

- Yawkey Family Inn at Children's Hospital Boston; Yawkey Foundations, 990 Washington Street, Suite 315, Dedham, MA 02026; Phone (781) 329-7470, email yawkey@yawkey.org

- Children's Flight of Hope, 1005 Dresser Court, Raleigh, NC 27609. https://www.childrensflightofhope.org

- Duke Children's Hospital, 300 W. Morgan Street, Suite 1200, Durham, NC 27701; Phone (919) 385-3138. Email dukekids@duke.edu

- Donate Life NC, PO Box 5536, Cary, NC 27512; Phone (919) 576-0615, https://www.do-natelifenc.org/ Register as an organ donor.

- The Make-A-Wish Foundation; Make-A-Wish America, Gift Processing, 1702 East Highland Ave., Suite 400, Phoenix, AZ 85016

- Disney World, Orlando, Florida

- Give Kids the World Village, 210 South Bass Road, Kissimmee, Fl 34746; https://www.gktw.org/

To Larry Leech II, my writing coach, you helped me, an untrained writer with a story to tell, write a book that's hopefully worth reading. I am forever grateful.

To cousin Monty Joynes and his wife Pat, thank you for the poem and copyediting. Your encouragement and love helped me finish this project.

To Alleghany Writers, our local writing group, your critique, advice, and encouragement kept me going. www.alleghanywriters.com

To Chuck Bingham, my running mentor and spiritual guide, God put you in my life when my family and I needed you. To Him be the glory.

To the many churches and hundreds, if not thousands, that prayed for Landon and our family, your love and prayers sustained us through this ordeal and continue to propel us forward.

To the hospitals and doctors, God gave you knowledge and ability. Through your hands, dedication, and compassionate care, Landon survived and continues to thrive.

To the many volunteers who gave time and money to "Make a Miracle for Landon." You did.

God Saved My Grandson.

Thank You.   *- Eldon Joines*

Made in the USA
Columbia, SC
13 July 2021

41619712R00163